PRIME

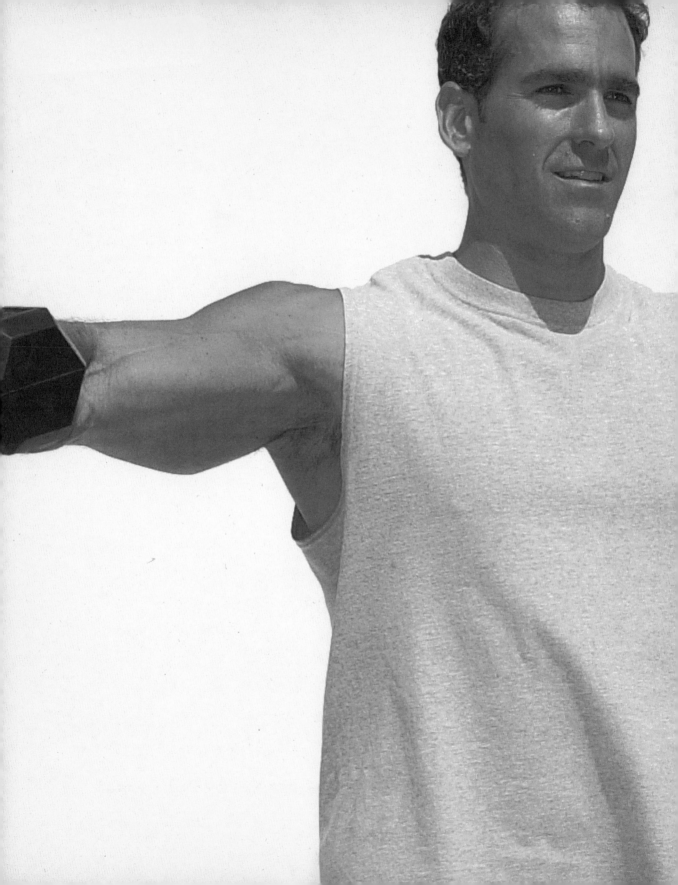

PRIME

THE COMPLETE GUIDE TO

Being Fit

Looking Good

Bob
Paris

Feeling Great

Photographs by Per Bernal

A PERIGEE BOOK

Most Perigee Books are available at special quantity discounts for bulk purchases for sales promotions, premiums, fund-raising, or educational use. Special books, or book excerpts, can also be created to fit specific needs.

For details, write: Special Markets, The Berkley Publishing Group, 375 Hudson Street, New York, New York 10014.

A Perigee Book
Published by The Berkley Publishing Group
A division of Penguin Putnam Inc.
375 Hudson Street
New York, New York 10014

FIRST EDITION: January 2002

Published simultaneously in Canada.

Visit our website at www.penguinputnam.com

LIBRARY OF CONGRESS CATALOGING-IN-PUBLICATION DATA

Paris, Bob.
Prime : the complete guide to being fit, looking good, feeling great / Bob Paris.
p. cm.
Includes index.
ISBN 0-399-52719-2
1. Health. 2. Exercise. 3. Nutrition. 4. Longevity. I. Title.

RA776 .P1835 2002
610—dc21   2001053108

Printed in the United States of America

10 9 8 7 6 5 4 3 2 1

For B. A. L.

And to the memory of my father

CONTENTS

FIRST THINGS FIRST

Procrastination of vital tasks is a close relative of incompetence and a handmaiden of inefficiency.

—R. ALEC MACKENZIE

I have spent nearly 20 years mastering, teaching, and practicing the knowledge I share in this book. That said, here is my first piece of advice:

Don't just skip to the workouts. Read the whole book first. The information contained in *Prime* may help you transform your fitness life.

I say this right from the start because, being a man myself, I can certainly identify with how the male mind sometimes works. When beginning a new project, a lot of men avoid reading tedious directions and throw themselves right into the "real work." Since getting into better shape can certainly be considered a self-improvement project, some guys would consider anything other than heading—gung-ho—straight into the workouts to be a waste of valuable time. This belief, however, leads many men to simply repeat the same flawed patterns over and over, rarely maximizing results, and perhaps doing little more than reinforcing a tremendously frustrating loop.

There is much more to getting into better shape than just doing the workouts. So, at the risk of belaboring my point, I will make this simple guarantee:

If you skip straight to the workouts and ignore the other stuff, your results will probably be a fraction of what they could be—that is, if you make any gains at all.

Also, if you're afraid that using the exercise information in *Prime* will lead you to become "muscle-bound," you can relax—nothing could be further from the truth. This is not a hard-core bodybuilding book. I place far less emphasis on building big muscles than I do on all other aspects of fitness and total wellness for the grown-up man. Besides, no one *accidentally* becomes muscle-bound. Building bodybuilder-style muscles takes years of dedicated and focused hard work. It isn't a condition easily stumbled upon, no matter what the old, outdated myths might say.

The advice in *Prime* revolves around creating a fitness plan to suit each man's individualized goals. Above all else, I'll emphasize learning to build new and better fitness habits that work both from the inside out and the outside in. I strive to teach balance and greater self-understanding. For many men, that can be a revolutionary concept. Therefore I should also begin *Prime* with this word of caution:

If you follow the advice in this book, you may, as a side effect of your efforts, build a rather nice body.

As you read *Prime*, I challenge you to reexamine your beliefs about what it means to be fit and how to go about getting there. Read this book as if you know little or nothing about exercise. In other words, read it with an open mind.

ACKNOWLEDGMENTS

Thank you to my publisher, John Duff, for his support of this project, and to Stuart Calderwood for his work as my editor.

My agents, Jan Miller and Michael Broussard, merit many thanks as well.

For his wonderful photographic contributions, I thank Per Bernal.

For his generous help with all matters technological, I thank Normand Halde.

And finally, for his incredible support and research, I thank Brian LeFurgey.

INTRODUCTION
For the Man Who Wasn't Born Yesterday

You cannot teach a man anything; you can only lead him to find it in himself.

—GALILEO

LOOK DEEPER

Most of the fitness books written for men focus on quick and easy fixes. There's a simple reason for that: People want fast change; they want it easy and they want it yesterday. People turn to fitness books with an almost desperate desire for quick and painless change of the outside "packaging" of their bodies. Since supply generally gravitates toward demand, most fitness books focus their entire energy on the outside "package"—slimmer waistlines, bigger biceps, and so forth.

Scores of new books are written each year that purport to give the reader the latest fast track to a washboard stomach or a ten-pound weight loss by exploiting some trendy, superficial gimmick; some effortless miracle.

Readers flock to the new trend, perhaps even experience a brief level of positive change, yet quickly discard this exciting new miracle breakthrough after a short time and fall back into the same old habits. Why does this happen? Because any fitness plan that focuses exclusively on surface issues (such as fast weight loss or rapid muscle gain) ignores the fact

PRIME

that positive change requires more than a gimmick. Real sustainable change requires one to work on the inside (the mind and spirit) as well as the outside (the physical body). Beyond that, real and sustainable self-improvement requires that the inside and the outside become interactive, with progress in one driving advances in the other.

In other words, when pursued in a healthy, balanced manner, a slimmer waistline will generally improve a man's self-image, just as a better self-image will help that man eat and exercise in healthy, balanced ways that will result in a slimmer waistline. The inside (self-regard) and the outside (the waistline) interact with and influence each other.

A fitness book's focus on quick, easy solutions to fitness problems (something along the lines of the old "lose twenty pounds in ten days" approach) cheats the reader out of discovering the deeper personal development that takes place when people take their fitness efforts beneath the superficiality of quick-fix gimmicks and into the true heart of interactive, genuine self-improvement.

THE REAL SOLUTION

There is so much confusion regarding what it takes to get and stay in shape. It's time for a new and better way of doing things; a way that transcends superficial methods.

True fitness doesn't come through temporarily losing twenty pounds. It comes from learning how to go about looking good, feeling great, being fit, and, perhaps most importantly, really and truly learning to respect ourselves inside and out.

When a man seeks true, long-lasting fitness goals—and not the transient, usually frustrating quick-fix goal of the moment—he allows his inside perspective to drive his outside actions, and vice versa. He learns how to truly take charge and become genuinely fit.

In *Prime*, I will place equal emphasis on both the package (muscles, fat, skin, hair, and so forth) and the contents (self-understanding, motivation, balance, et cetera). I will do my best to encourage you to do so as well.

THE GROWN-UP MAN

The overwhelming majority of fitness books written for men are not only directed toward quick fixes, but also seem geared toward 20-somethings or (to a lesser degree) senior citizens. What about all the guys who are in between those two age groups? There certainly doesn't seem to be much quality information about the mid-life changes in the male body and how they relate to getting and staying in shape.

So, I set out to write a book that would act as a tool to help guide what I like to call the *grown-up man* (who is technically neither young nor old) toward putting his own unique fitness needs firmly on track.

In this book I want to totally demystify the step-by-step process that you, as a grown-up man, can use to feel and look your best, whether you are approaching 40 or have passed it. It should be noted that for the sake of simplicity, throughout the book I'll refer to this grown-up man as the *40+ man*, and those of you who are only approaching that magic line in the cultural sand and haven't yet turned 40 shouldn't read that as a message that this book isn't for you. It is. Your age as you begin a *Prime* program will be as individual as your strategy for positive change will be.

Prime is for the man who finds himself in a new or different phase in life: a phase in which the easy assumptions of youth have faded away, yet the realistic desire for an amazing, fit, and active life still burns.

Prime is for the man willing to face, with open eyes and mind, the reality that while the body he lives in might basically be the same one that he spent his twenties in, its needs at mid-life—especially regarding staying fit and slowing the aging process to a snail's pace—have evolved. And evolution can be a thing of great beauty, something to be both embraced and celebrated. We simply must develop an effective strategy for directing this evolution toward positive outcomes.

Prime is, beyond everything else, a guide for the grown-up man seeking a course of informed, intelligent action, directed toward true, deep self-improvement.

I ask that you approach the information, philosophies, and programs in *Prime* willing to participate in a positive way in your own evolution.

CREATING CHANGE

Throughout this book I'll address strategies for accepting the changes that are beyond our control, integrated with a step-by-step plan for taking charge and transforming the parts of ourselves that—with informed effort—can be changed and improved.

You'll also notice that, although *Prime* is very structured in its philosophy and routines, it also encourages a high level of individuality in putting the various concepts to work. That's important. We each have a unique path, and there are no cookie-cutter solutions. You certainly won't find any here. The history and details of your fitness life (or lack of it) are completely your own. I want to help you discover ways to maximize the individualized goals that you set while reading this book.

TRUST ME, I UNDERSTAND

The advice and routines you'll read about here are simply guidelines culled from my own lifetime of experience in the fitness field. I have also faced (and still face) many of the same issues I'll address in this book in my own struggle to allow my fitness philosophies and practices to grow and evolve with age. Just because I look a certain way in the pictures in this book doesn't mean that I don't understand the process you may be going through. I don't necessarily find any of the concepts I discuss here any easier or more automatic than you do. In a way, I'm writing this book both for you and myself, because I—like you—want my middle years to be as good as or better than what came before. I seek, just as you seek, ways to be truly fit, look good, and feel great during life's prime years.

TIME FLIES

A little while ago I was a boy. You were too. Remember? Now, suddenly the years seem to pass with the relative speed that months or weeks did in childhood. Older people always told us that it would happen that way, right? So here we stand inside these bodies that might barely resemble our 20-year-old selves, living out habits that only seem to make matters worse. What can we do about it? The answer to that question is one of the primary reasons this book exists.

It doesn't take the Fed chairman to realize that we live in a rapidly changing world, with enormous leaps in technology, medicine, and other types of practical knowledge unfolding before our eyes. Yet in spite of all these changes, if we live with our eyes open to the world and possess some sense of curiosity, we still seek answers to some very basic human questions.

JUST THE FACTS

Now, I would never claim to be able to offer anything other than my own observations and opinions regarding many of the complex questions raised by technological advances, and I doubt that you're reading this book to get my take on many of these issues. However, I have observed that while new advances in technology and medicine may support us, confuse us, and both simplify and complicate our lives, there remains one extraordinarily complex technology that each of us lives with every day, one which, if we learn to understand and use it properly, can be the most wondrous personal-development tool ever invented. What is this amazing technology? Look in a mirror. It's you.

The combined elements of your own unique, individualized body—from the muscles that hang off your skeleton, to the thoughts that bang around your brain; from your perceptions to your heartbeat—constitute the most amazing personal-development tool on the planet.

"Yeah, right," you might say, "I'm forty-five, totally stressed out, my back aches . . . and what the hell does this gut of mine have to do with personal development?"

Stick with me and I'll show you.

CHANGING TIMES

At the beginning of the twentieth century, the average American male lived to be about 45 years old. These days, that same average man might well expect to live past 75. So, even if you end up living an average lifespan and you've hit forty-some (follow my complex math here), you know that you're just beyond halfway through your life. Even if you're in your 50s and are merely average (life-expectancy-wise), you still have decades ahead of you.

Bearing that in mind, I'd like you to take a few seconds and try to recall how long your life has felt so far, from your first memory up until this moment. Now, try to briefly recall everything that's taken place in your life just during the last twenty years. Probably seems like a lifetime in itself, right? Imagine, though, if your next twenty years are just as full as the preceding twenty, how much life you can fit into them.

I find it rather comforting to know that during the next twenty years, I can take what I've learned from the last twenty and make intelligent choices that help me continue to grow as a man. That's one of the beauties of passing time.

Of course, there is another reality that goes hand in hand with passing time. Like the old cliché about time speeding up as we get older, the one about the aging body going downhill fast may have sneaked up on you, too. Even if the fulfillment of that particular cliché didn't really surprise you, if you're like me, you must at least occasionally be shocked to come face-to-face with the stark reality that everything does change. Most of these changes aren't the sorts of things we'd put on our Christmas wish list, either: wrinkles, fat, hairs either magically appearing or disappearing, but not where we want them; it goes on and on.

So, what's a (former) boy to do? Panic? Get ticked off? Pretend nothing's happening until you're eventually standing in that bright tunnel of light we hear so much about? I suppose you could make those choices, but it doesn't seem like much of a solution, does it?

There is a better way. But let's take first things first. You and I must realize one simple thing: We aren't kids anymore, and there's nothing we can do about it. Comb-overs won't change it. Red convertibles and young lovers won't, either. We simply have to face facts. Our bodies are aging. We can't control that.

But here's the good news: While many of the various changes that come with aging are inevitable, we can also exercise enormous control over not only how those changes happen, but perhaps more importantly, how we respond to them.

Just as the average life span is increasing well beyond what our ancestors faced, the quality of our aging process doesn't have to be the same as theirs either. People are proving that every day. They are refusing to simply, passively assign themselves to the psychological, physical, and spiritual old-folks' home just because some certain birthday has come and gone.

On the other hand, even with an expanding life expectancy, huge numbers of men may be living longer, but the quality of their lives, particularly regarding health, declines with each passing year. There is a simple reason for this: Most men die from how they choose to live.

Many of us have accumulated habits over the years that—even if we outlive our ancestors—dramatically reduce the quality of the second half of our lives. In fact, many of us might spend much of the second half of life battling a broad array of health obstacles (such as heart disease, obesity, and various forms of cancer) brought about by our own unhealthy choices. And that is what we want to get at.

We don't want to simply reshape the body; we want to make better choices. We want to break free of old, entrenched habits that harm our lives. We want to reject passively allowing ourselves to decline without a fight simply because we aren't "young" anymore.

Throughout this book I will encourage you to embrace your current age and condition. I want to help you discover your own ability to create dynamic goals and empowered actions on your own behalf—not as a denial of aging, but rather as a welcoming of new possibilities.

Our lives can be more profound and glorious than ever, but it won't be because we've found quicker or easier ways to build big, strong muscles or lose a gut. Those things are great and they're certainly wonderful goals (if indeed they turn out to be your own individual goals), but beyond those physical things, I believe that with the information I provide you in

Prime and with your own fully conscious effort and self-directed wisdom, you will discover a part of yourself that you might never even have known you possess.

You may learn body pride for the first time in your life. You may discover what it means to really like the way you're put together. You may learn to embrace the unchangeable aspects about yourself that you see as flawed, and you might also learn to change a few things that you do have control over. You may transform your health. You may do all these things and more, if you will allow me to gently transform the way you look at exercise, wellness, nutrition, and much, much more.

You don't need to abandon the idea that you can look and feel great just because you're 40 or older. It is never, ever too late to create positive change in your life. Anyone who tells you otherwise is a fool. No matter what your age, you can improve the way you feel and the way you feel about yourself. You can look better and maximize the best health possible. *You can do that.*

To do it though, you may have to make some changes in how you look at things. You may need to totally reprogram the way you see yourself, the way you think about your body, and the way you treat it. Perhaps you've been conditioned to believe that the decline that comes after your late 20s or early 30s is inevitable. It isn't. But to make sure that it isn't, you're going to have to learn how to really care *about* yourself. That, my friend, is the only truly effective, long-lasting way to learn how to take better care *of* yourself.

Sometimes talking about really caring about ourselves—truly learning to love our own bodies and so forth—makes men uncomfortable. It seems to smack of some kind of "boomer" angst or perhaps an unhealthy self-absorption. That's not what *Prime* is about. It is instead dedicated to helping grown-up men redefine, in a balanced way, what individualized self-care truly means. *Prime* is an effective tool for helping 40+ men develop step-by-step programs that will build fitness and wellness levels equal to or greater than they've had at any other time in their lives.

What should you expect from *Prime*? The truest answer to that question will come from you. But here is my promise: I can direct you; provide information, blueprints, and guidance; and bring to the table all of my 20 years of experience and knowledge. You will decide what to do with it: either encounter it and turn away, or go deeply into it and transform the quality of your life.

I do, however, want to give you an idea of the results you can expect if you follow the advice in this book and adjust it with honesty and integrity to your own unique life, circumstances and goals:

By using *Prime*, you can expect to:

1. Improve lean muscle mass and tone

2. Decrease body fat and keep it controllable

3. Instill a balanced, healthy approach to food and nutritional supplements

4. Learn to respect the unchangeable but uniquely personal aspects of your body

5. Develop a plan of action for changing those things that can be changed

6. Evolve toward exercise habits that work for your individualized goals

7. Change old habits that no longer serve your fitness life

8. Put in place a self-care system for your skin, hair, and appearance that helps you look your best

9. Learn to understand the balance between desired outcome and willingness to invest effort

10. Balance your fitness goals so you'll feel great on the inside and look fantastic on the outside

Prime is about helping grown-up men discover ways to live their lives fully and health-fully. It is about positive change of a kind that will exceed superficiality and go deeply into the way a man feels, and the way he feels about himself.

That sort of change doesn't come free. It isn't necessarily easy. And it sure isn't going to happen by accident. But if you stay with me through each chapter of this book, I can promise that your outlook toward what is possible in your life can be transformed. I can help you to learn to use the amazing technology of your body to create a self-strengthening cycle of positive change, both inside and out.

I should be honest with you right up front. The approach I take in *Prime* will not allow you much passivity. After all, you aren't some innocent bystander in your own life. You control it. You create the reality of your life with each choice you make. The philosophies and programs in *Prime* will primarily revolve around helping you make more informed, healthier choices.

What I'm talking about isn't some late-night infomercial, quickie gimmick that'll leave you feeling ripped off and worse than ever. I believe in a full-blown, inside-out and outside-in, active approach, because taking such broad-based action on your own behalf changes you in ways that exceed fat reduction, muscle tone, and lower cholesterol.

> *Dare to be yourself.*
> —ANDRÉ GIDE

LOOK INSIDE

Prime is a full-participation experience, especially since creating tremendous positive change requires an evolution in belief, thought, and most of all, action. Positive change also requires you to make active choices.

I believe that we are the sum total of our choices in life. So, I'll lead you off with a choice:

Imagine that you stand today facing two doors. One door leads into your life (and for the sake of this example, your fitness life in particular) as it exists right now, and this path extends out toward the horizon along the same trajectory. By walking through the first door you continue to do everything the same way: You take the same actions (or inactions). You eat the same, exercise the same, care for yourself the same. Now factor in the continuing aging process. What will the results be in a year, five years, ten years into the future?

The second door leads to a road less traveled. And here's a secret: Only you can know what that road actually looks like; only you can walk it. I can give you a map and compass. I can help you learn how to use them. We can talk about the lay of the land; discuss both the hazards and the paradises. But once you step through that door, you will put into motion changes that will improve your life and will continue improving it, so long as you stay aware and keep making self-respecting, responsible choices to take good care of yourself; so long as you continue to participate positively in your own evolution.

GO AFTER YOUR DREAMS

If you're reading this book—whether it was given to you by someone who cares or you picked it out yourself—that simple action likely means that you want to walk through that second door. Go inside yourself, take a good, hard look, and, as a grown-up man, decide to reclaim (or claim for the first time) your own body, health, and well being, so that you might enter into the next phase of your adult life in better shape and more in control of your life's quality than ever before.

Are you ready? Are you ready to come into the prime years of your life stronger, healthier, more confident, more centered, happier, and more in charge of your fitness life?

Then come with me into the world of *Prime*.

PRIME

PART ONE

STOP THE CLOCK

When you think all is lost, the future remains.
—ROBERT H. GODDARD

AS A MAN 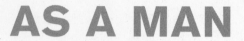 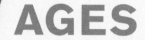AGES

In our culture, with each passing year of the average man's life, his physical activity decreases significantly. As a man ages—and especially once he's reached 40—he's begun to rapidly lose muscle strength, tone, and size, and his body fat steadily increases. The reasons for these changes are simultaneously simple and complex.

Many of the changes can be attributed to the way our bodies are wired—what they were essentially designed to do. To understand this, take a quick look back in time, before technology replaced physicality.

Life in the old days was tough. Our ancestors lived to an average age of 45 and generally spent many of those years toiling at some difficult manual labor. Their lives were so brutally active that most of us would crumble if suddenly subjected to such a grueling physical workload.

Given the relative ease of our modern culture, most of us have a difficult time imagining what life must have been like prior to the innovations that we now take for granted. Few of us perform anything close to the sort of manual labor that was previously such an entrenched part of daily reality—everything from hunting for food to clearing woodlands with an axe—both to get the wood for a cabin to live in and to create crop-fields that had to be tended by hand.

In fact, our modern lives are so non-physical that few of us can even imagine getting up off the couch and crossing the room to change TV channels, much less having to plow a field by hand. Yet, to put it into vastly oversimplified terms, this is what our bodies were designed to do.

Now, don't get me wrong: I'm not saying that to be in shape, we must return to the good old days of a hundred years ago. Yes, our ancestors used their bodies more in their day-to-day lives, but they also died young (by our standards) because of the hard lives they led. This is the ironic part of all of our modern medical and technological advances. On average, we live a lot longer, but most of us are pretty sluggish, if not downright sedentary. This in turn harms our health during the second half of our expanded years. We have lengthened our life spans, but simultaneously reduced their overall physical quality.

SLOWING DOWN

In addition to the technological advances that have subtracted physicality from our everyday survival, there are other bodily factors that simply shift with age. For example, after we reach a certain maturity level, the production of hormones—such as testosterone and various other complex growth factors—that fuel our muscles goes into decline. Because we are no longer growing (maturing through puberty), our metabolic rates slow. Muscle mass decreases just as fat accumulation increases. And it isn't just inactivity and the biology of aging that cause this shift.

There's also this modern diet that many of us survive on by eating, for no better reason than that we imagine it to be convenient. Because of a perception of short-term convenience, we keep eating it, and, of course, with enough repetition and time, the bad diet (like any activity) becomes a nearly insurmountable force of habit.

After simple hard-wiring and the sedentary lifestyle that's evolved out of an era of technological advances, poor nutrition is perhaps the greatest driving force behind the 40+ man's developing health problems. Habits of convenience, by-products of the same advances that enable us to live longer, develop into seemingly unbreakable patterns that continue for no better reason than that we don't stop to consider the consequences or the alternatives.

SUPER-SIZE IT

Think about it: Do you really believe that you can eat a daily diet that revolves around double cheeseburgers (and the like), live in a mostly sedentary way, and still age well? Even if you've gotten away with it throughout your 20s and 30s, by the time you hit 40, the bill is going to come due.

With time and age, we get ourselves into loops of behaviors and beliefs that become stubbornly self-reinforcing. For example: Let's say that you do survive by eating junk food because its convenient, but it makes you feel lousy. Feeling lousy, and through force of habit, you figure "What the hell," and eat more junk food, making yourself feel worse—in a continuous loop. Can you see how that works?

It doesn't have to be that way, though. With only minor changes in your thoughts, beliefs, and actions, you can change any bad habit. But before you can alter any established pattern, you must first identify it.

Let me illustrate another example of a typical loop that a 40+ man in our culture might get caught up in. See if you can identify with any of this loop of behavior and belief:

- A man finds himself physically inactive because all he seems to do in life is get up, go to work, come home, watch TV, go to bed, and repeat the same cycle day after day.

- Because of decades of this sort of inactivity—along with the hormonal changes inevitable with passing 40—lean muscle mass goes into sharp decline.

- Inactivity and a slowing metabolism cause a gain in body fat, which only grows more stubborn each year.

- Decades of having eaten what's easy, fast, and convenient (but almost never truly healthy) contribute to quicker fat accumulation and the beginnings of health problems such as high cholesterol.

- Seeing the muscles dwindle and fat grow, the man develops a complacent attitude toward exercise and good eating, and this attitude gets reinforced, developing into the "why bother" syndrome.

- Long-standing dislike of various physical characteristics, combined with a feeling of having become shut off from his body, reinforce the man's avoidance of anything too involved with concentrating on declining fitness and health.

- When considering health and fitness (or a growing gut), the man hopes that some effortless miracle is going to come along any minute and change everything.

- Because the man has gotten so far out of shape and has essentially developed the attitude that avoidance is the best strategy, his outward appearance begins to decline, and he tells himself that this change is simply inevitable.

- This leads him right back to the beginning: a life built around inactivity and decline.

There is a far better way, a path of health and wellness that fights against this tide of a decline that seems inevitable, yet doesn't have to happen at all—if you're willing to take charge. And that's what the rest of this book is all about.

Don't be discouraged if you feel caught in one of these loops. It's never too late to begin taking good care of yourself. You can turn your fitness life around starting today. First, let me tell you a little bit about my own journey through these same issues. Then we'll get you on the road to your *Prime*.

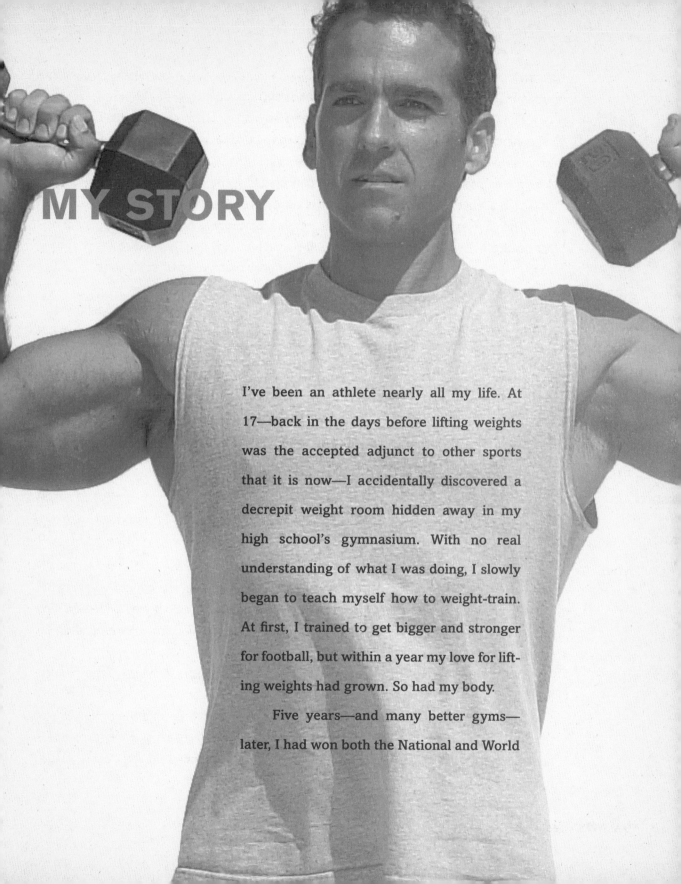

MY STORY

I've been an athlete nearly all my life. At 17—back in the days before lifting weights was the accepted adjunct to other sports that it is now—I accidentally discovered a decrepit weight room hidden away in my high school's gymnasium. With no real understanding of what I was doing, I slowly began to teach myself how to weight-train. At first, I trained to get bigger and stronger for football, but within a year my love for lifting weights had grown. So had my body.

Five years—and many better gyms—later, I had won both the National and World

Championships in the sport of bodybuilding. I went on to have a very successful professional career until I retired from competition at the age of 31.

Throughout my competitive years, my exercise and diet habits were driven by immediate, concrete, competitive goals. I weight-trained to build muscle. I ate well and did cardio exercises to keep my fat down. I stretched to avoid injuries that could take my career off-track. I kept myself motivated, aware, and firmly connected to all the various systems of my athletic life. As a side effect of all this goal-oriented effort, I stayed in great shape, both inside and out.

Then my goals went through a dramatic shift. Since I was no longer competing, I neither needed nor wanted to maintain the 230-pound physique that required so many intense hours in the gym. My workouts grew sporadic. After so many years of strict nutrition, it also seemed easier to eat anything I craved—so I did.

I found it difficult to make a transition from the all-out intensity of my competitive routines to a lower-key, more balanced approach. In a way, I surrendered to the inevitability of living a life without exercise and good nutrition.

My body changed. I was fortunate enough to have a great metabolism, so I didn't get visibly overweight, but my muscle mass dwindled and under my shirt—where I once had champion abdominals—pockets of fat were slowly sneaking up on me. My joints ached from not being as active. My cholesterol rose. I could no longer go out and run five miles on a whim without nearly collapsing. My self-image suffered, but in an indirect way: I simply stopped thinking about my body. This doesn't sound all that profound at first, but by ignoring it so completely, I was giving myself permission not to care. Regarding my body and overall health, I had gone from being completely proactive to merely drifting along, resting on my metabolic laurels.

In a perverse way, my great metabolism was cheating me. By remaining essentially lean even while fairly sedentary, I was able to fool myself into believing that I was in better shape than I really was. This went on for several years, but I contented myself with the notion that life was good and that I'd earned time away from having my focus revolve around my fitness needs.

Then 40 started coming my way. My great metabolism began to fail me, almost imperceptibly at first, but then it really began to slow down.

My father died of a sudden heart attack at the age of 64. Beyond the overwhelming shock of the loss lay thoughts of my own eventual mortality. His death also made me take a hard look at how I was taking care of myself and how, if I continued along the same passive road, I would pay a heavy price down the line. It was time for a change.

I went back through the stacks of training journals that I'd kept over the years, and began, as I'd done many times before, with a plan. I wanted the plan to be simple and easy to use. I wanted it to fit into my busy life, but in a way that helped me evolve to the next level of great health.

I knew that I didn't want to be huge; I wanted to be in great shape. I wanted to take control of my aging process. I got busy with putting my new plan to work. The results were amazing.

In twelve weeks, using principles that I outline in this book, I transformed my body and my outlook. My muscles grew strong, lean and flexible. I learned to love eating well and to take great care of myself—not out of vanity, but because I was worth the effort.

Best of all, I found that I didn't need to dedicate hours every day to my new habits. My training sessions took no more than an hour each day—usually less. And once the habit was formed, it was just as easy to make nutritious meals as it was to grab something that wasn't good for my health. I loved the way my skin looked when I took care of it; I loved the way I felt and felt about myself. In fact, I felt better, in every possible way, at 40 than I had at 25. That wouldn't be true if I hadn't been willing to take a good, hard look at my habits and make informed and intelligent adjustments.

This was definitely not the hard-core approach that I'd grown so accustomed to in the past. There was, however, a valuable lesson in balance for me. It's a lesson that I want to share with you throughout this book: Just because you are 40 or older—and no matter what your experience level with fitness has been—you can break free of old destructive habits and find a new and better way. I hope that this lesson becomes a discovery just as transforming for you as it has been for me.

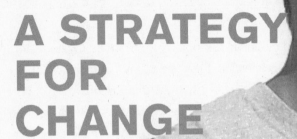

A STRATEGY
FOR
CHANGE

There are several essential truths that a man must face as he begins the road toward changing his fitness life beyond the age of 40:

1. He lives inside a body that is uniquely individual and in a constant state of change.

2. He must fully accept the reality of those aspects of himself that can be changed and those that cannot.

3. His physical body will quickly deteriorate if it isn't used, and it will also require greater rest and maintenance.

4. More exercise is not necessarily better, but none is even worse.

5.   When the easy fitness of youth has passed, he will benefit from his fitness investment in exact proportion to the intelligent effort he puts in.

6.   Having established long-standing habits, he can't be compelled to take care of himself. If he doesn't want to eat right or exercise, he will find every imaginable excuse not to do so.

7.   He will almost never take charge of his fitness life until he must. He can only hope that he will decide his fate before circumstances decide for him.

You see, throughout your life you have created either passive-or active-change goals for yourself. A passive-change goal would be eating a terrible diet and being as active as a hibernating bear. An active-change goal would be something like beginning a low-fat diet and a light workout routine after many sedentary years.

What we're going to do in *Prime* is get you to decide for yourself not just to take charge of your change-oriented goals, but also to take intelligent action to achieve them.

RISING TO THE OCCASION

It is essential to remember that in addition to the changes that will simply come your way, you are making choices each day about your quality of life. I'm certainly not saying that you must have nice muscles and a trim waist to have a good life, but if you had those things, don't you think you'd be happier? Maybe yes, maybe no. I say that because one thing that I've learned from my own experience is that being in great physical shape, in and of itself, will not make you happy.

Does it sound as if I am contradicting myself? I'm not. You *should* strive to get into better shape, but not because you think that being buffed will solve all your problems. It won't. The problems of life will still come. Being in great shape, however, will help you be in the physical and mental condition to deal with the complexities of life in a far better way. How? Imagine two different scenarios with these conditions: You live on the coast and a severe hurricane is headed toward your house.

In the first scenario, you're over 40, and you've lived on junk food and sat on your couch for so long that the backs of your legs have the pattern of the material etched in them like tattoos. Are you able to take the immediate physical actions necessary to get your home and family ready to face the coming storm?

Now imagine that you're totally fit, and the same storm is coming your way. Can you see how you could take immediate physical action—kick totally into high gear—and bring all your self-created strength, stamina, and mental focus to bear on the situation as you rose to what needed to be done?

Which scenario do you want your life to be like?

INSIDE AND OUT

The happiness and fulfillment that your *Prime* levels of fitness bring to your life will come from inside you. That is where true lifelong fitness begins. I want to help you understand that all of your efforts toward taking charge of change in your life should focus on you, not as an assorted bunch of body parts or fat molecules, but as a whole man.

While it is essential to work on your physical fitness, you should also balance that with the way you view yourself and the way you respond to the health issues that come with age.

Here are two important questions to ask yourself. Be honest in answering them, too. If you aren't, you're the only person you'll be fooling.

- ■ What do you want to get out of your investment in pursuing better health and fitness?

- ■ How much time and effort are you willing to commit, on an ongoing basis, to those desires?

Now hang on to those answers. They are going to be important as you start out on the road to reclaiming your *Prime*. They're also only the first of a series of questions that I'm going to get you to ask yourself. There are many more coming up that will help you get the most out of your invested efforts with this book.

Before we get to that, though, I'm going to share with you one of my favorite formulas for creating positive change in your life. I use it myself—especially with my new approach to fitness—and it has literally helped me work miracles in transformation.

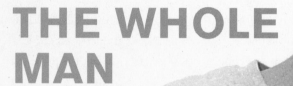

THE WHOLE MAN

Your body is a system in which each part directly influences the others. Your perceptions about one part of yourself will likely dictate what you do with the other parts. For example, if you've always viewed yourself as unathletic, your actions probably reflect that. You may not exercise or pay much attention to the quality of your nutrition, and that leads your muscles to shrink and your fat cells to grow, furthering your perception of yourself as unathletic. If these are lifelong perceptions and actions, by the time you reach 40 they are fairly well entrenched, and you're going to need a step-by-step plan for creating change. That is *Prime*'s main focus.

In addition to developing change strategies, we'll be building an understanding that the best possible fitness plans focus on balancing and improving all the various elements of the whole man.

Remember that in *Prime*, we're reaching to exceed the surface solutions that focus exclusively on fat loss or muscle building, striving instead to find the healthy, well-rounded, grown-up guy inside of us all. We'll need a system that allows us to see and understand just how interactive the various parts of our minds and bodies are when we're developing strategies for balanced change.

There are three general areas of balanced focus that go into developing great fitness and health. Each one stands on its own as a worthy area of focus and effort, yet they also blend together and interact, helping to create spectacular levels of wellness for the whole man.

The *three key areas of focus* are:

1. Motivated mind

2. Fit body

3. Sound nutrition

Each of these *three key areas of focus* is a rather broad category. After all, there are many elements that go into developing a MOTIVATED MIND or a FIT BODY. In future sections, I will provide an expanded, in-depth look at how each of these *three key areas of focus* is comprised of several additional and important aspects.

NO JARGON

I don't have the audacity to claim that *Prime* will present you with all the answers you seek. I can only present you with one path, created from my own philosophies, experiences, and understanding. I believe that it's a great way to get what you're looking for. The information that I share in this book won't contain lots of quotations from medical studies or other scientific mumbo-jumbo. I believe in a well-informed approach, but I find that using lots of outside source materials tends to confuse matters. Instead, I present commonsense answers for the everyday man who is looking for a no-nonsense road to better health and fitness.

I'M NOT A DOCTOR

You may have also noticed that I did not include a specific category for HEALTH, even though this is one of the primary concerns for the 40+ man who is launching this kind of program. There are plenty of developing health issues facing the 40+ man, such as heart disease, obesity, diabetes, and cancer (among many others). If any of these are issues in your life, you must consult your doctor. I'm in no position to deliver specific medical advice. In *Prime*, I can only offer advice related to motivation, fitness, nutrition, and appearance. I will add, however, that many of the major medical issues that begin to surface as a man ages can be addressed (without neglecting sound, consistent medical advice) through proper diet and exercise and a motivated, positive mental outlook. Improving your habits can change your long-term health.

SO SEE YOUR DOCTOR

Here's an amazing fact: One-third of American men haven't had a medical checkup in the past year, and nine million haven't seen a doctor in the past five years.

It is often said that prevention is the key to a healthy life. Well, it certainly is one of them—and yet most men take better care of their cars than they do of their own bodies. Like a fine automobile, the human body also needs regular "tune-ups." If we hear a strange rattle coming from under the hood, we'll take our car to the local garage and have a mechanic diagnose the problem, and yet, as men, we often ignore our bodies when we feel chest pains, or experience dizziness, shortness of breath, or some other sign that something could be wrong. Why? It's most likely a blend of fear, denial, and guys' tendency to "tough it out." And yet by being proactive, paying attention to and respecting early warning signs, and having scheduled "tune-ups"—instead of only seeing the doctor when that annoying chest pain becomes a first heart attack—we can prevent a medical emergency or catastrophe.

Did You Know?

The leading causes of death for men are:

1. Heart attack

2. Cancer (lung, prostate, colorectal)

3. Accidents (car wrecks, guns, drowning, fire)

4. Stroke

5. Obstructive lung disease

6. Pneumonia and influenza

7. HIV infection

8. Suicide

9. Diabetes

10. Homicide

While we aren't usually able to control things like accidents and homicide, the rest of the list above sure lends itself to making modifications in personal behavior, especially when early detection and a preventive, healthy lifestyle can save your life.

If you are having difficulty understanding why a positive change in lifestyle is important to the 40+ man, here are a few rather startling statistics for you:

- One in five men can expect to die of heart disease before the age of 75.

- This year alone, twenty-three thousand men will die of colon cancer.

- Stroke is the leading cause of serious long-term disability, and more than sixty thousand men will die because of it this year.

- More than ninety thousand men will die of smoking-related illness this year.

- Thirty thousand men will die of prostate cancer this year.

THE PHYSICAL

The traditional annual exams of the past are not really considered necessary for most healthy adults. However, regular medical tests are necessary for early detection and treatment of many of the diseases mentioned in the list above. The chart below is a guideline for healthy men at average risk. (Those in poor health or considered "at risk" might require specific screenings more regularly.)

FREQUENCY	AGE 20–39	FREQUENCY	AGE 40–49	FREQUENCY	AGE 50+
MONTHLY	Skin self-exam, testicular self-exam	MONTHLY	Skin self-exam, testicular self-exam	MONTHLY	Skin self-exam, testicular self-exam
EVERY 2 YEARS	Blood pressure	EVERY YEAR	Skin exam	EVERY YEAR	Skin exam; fecal occult blood test, digital rectal exam (for prostate cancer), prostate-specific antigen (PSA) test
EVERY 3 YEARS	Skin exam	EVERY 2 YEARS	Blood pressure	EVERY 2 YEARS	Blood pressure
EVERY 5 YEARS	Cholesterol (total and HDL)	EVERY 3 YEARS	Fasting plasma glucose test (for diabetes)	EVERY 3 YEARS	Fasting plasma glucose test (for diabetes)
VARIABLE	HIV exam, eye exam (at least once before 40)	EVERY 5 YEARS	Cholesterol (total and HDL)	EVERY 5 YEARS	Cholesterol (total and HDL; this test every 3–5 years if over 65)
IMMUNIZATION	Tetanus booster (every 10 years), Hepatitis B once if at risk	VARIABLE	HIV exam, eye exam	EVERY 5 TO 10 YEARS	Colorectal cancer tests
		IMMUNIZATION	Tetanus booster (every 10 years), Hepatitis B once if at risk	VARIABLE	HIV exam, eye exam (this test every 1–2 years if over 65)
				IMMUNIZATION	Tetanus booster (every 10 years), influenza vaccine (yearly if over 65), pneumococcal vaccine (once after 65), Hepatitis B once if at risk

AND THEN THERE'S CHOLESTEROL

A couple of decades ago, there weren't many doctors who paid much attention to cholesterol. Times have clearly changed since the discovery of the direct link between cholesterol and heart disease.

Cholesterol is a soft, waxy substance found among the lipids (fats) in the bloodstream and in all your body's cells. It plays an important part in maintaining a healthy body: it's used to form cell membranes, certain hormones, and other necessary tissue. However, because cholesterol doesn't dissolve in blood, high levels play a major role in coronary heart disease, which in turn can lead to a heart attack.

LDL, or low-density lipoprotein, is known as the "bad" cholesterol. Too much LDL cholesterol can build up in the walls of the arteries that feed the heart and brain, thereby increasing the risk for heart disease. A low level of LDL cholesterol is desirable, as it indicates lower risk of heart attack.

HDL, or high-density lipoprotein, is called the "good" cholesterol because medical experts believe that it carries cholesterol away from arteries and back to the liver, where it is passed through the body. A high level of HDL cholesterol seems to protect against heart attack. (Conversely, low HDL levels are undesirable as they can increase risk.)

We get cholesterol in two ways: The liver produces varying amounts daily, and the rest comes from the food we eat. In theory, our body makes all the cholesterol that we need to keep us healthy, so we don't need to consume any. In addition to high blood cholesterol (high total and LDL levels), other heart-disease risk factors that every 40+ man should be aware of are smoking, physical inactivity, obesity, high blood pressure, low HDL cholesterol, diabetes, and family history of early heart attack.

The latest guidelines for cholesterol levels from the *National Cholesterol Education Program* are as follows:

TOTAL CHOLESTEROL	LDL (BAD) CHOLESTEROL	HDL (GOOD) CHOLESTEROL
Below 200: desirable	Below 100: optimal	Below 40: low
200–239: borderline high	100–129: near/above optimal	60 or above: high
240 or above: high	130–159: borderline high	
	160–189: high	
	190 or above: very high	

AND FINALLY, A WORD ABOUT SMOKING

If you've reached the age of 40 and you still smoke, I have one simple word of advice for you: QUIT.

Not exactly an original thought, I realize. But if you want to have any degree of good health in your life, you *must* find a way to stop inflicting upon yourself one of the culture's leading pathways to disease, ill health, and excruciating death.

I know that quitting is hard. Do you think I couldn't understand this because I'm a former athlete? You'd be wrong. I stole my first cigarette from my father's pack when I was twelve, and then I smoked all through my teens and into my early twenties (in spite of being an athlete). Yes, nicotine got its insidious claws into me. Yes, it was very, very hard to quit. And yes, I've gone back a couple of times during periods of personal hardship. But I found a way to quit, and you can too. If you don't, chances are it'll get you. We know too much about it now to deny that very basic fact. I don't care if you had (or know someone who had) a grandpa who smoked three packs a day and lived to 102. Some people also win the lottery.

Approach quitting as a recovering alcoholic approaches staying off booze: one day at a time. Just as the recovering alcoholic frequently hurts loved ones before getting sober, when you become a recovering smoker you will see clearly that you, too, were severely harming someone you should care deeply about: yourself. Quit today.

FIVE SIMPLE SECRETS
OF SELF-IMPROVEMENT

KEYS TO PERSONAL HAPPINESS

Are you pleased with how your body looks and feels right now? Have the years begun to catch up with you? If so, you must find an efficient way to take charge.

To take charge of those aspects of your life that are within your control, you can't just fire shots in the dark. Not if you want to maximize results. When you get past 40, you don't want to waste your time chasing an elusive target. You want your efforts to pay off.

You need an effective strategy.

FIVE SIMPLE SECRETS

Any plan for taking charge of effective change has two essential core ingredients:

It must be *personalized*, and it must be about *action*.

Any plan that's going to work efficiently—and keep working over the long haul—should take these two basic things into account and help you to:

1. Decide what it is you want and how it fits into your *personalized* needs;

2. Take strong, fact-based *action* to get what you want, and then make continual informed adjustments.

To fully capitalize on the first step, I suggest that you build a *personal profile* on yourself. You've got to know not just what it is that you want to focus on, but also what you already believe about it, and what your personal history is in relation to it.

To utilize the second step, you'll develop an *action plan*, working to gather all the facts you can about what you want, and then putting those facts to work in an organized and motivated way. Again, you should observe your progress and make adjustments.

Taking both of these important aspects into account, I've developed my own personal strategy for creating positive change. I've broken it down into five steps, with the first two involving a *personal profile* and the next three involving an *action plan*.

I call these my *five simple secrets of self-improvement*. You're going to be using these *five simple secrets* throughout this book. They are:

1. **IDENTIFY THE NEED:** Be able to name and describe the situation you seek to take charge of changing—in other words, the habits or behaviors that you want to go away from.

2. **ESTABLISH YOUR PERSPECTIVE:** In accordance with this specific need, ask yourself a series of guided questions, taking into consideration your own experience regarding the issue at hand, therefore establishing your individual point of view.

3. **GATHER THE FACTS:** Regarding the need at hand, seek out as much intelligent information as you can possibly find, and decide what applies to your individual situation.

4. **GO TO WORK:** Based on the facts and your unique perspective, set individualized strategies, and then take immediate and intelligent action directed toward the need.

5. **MAKE SMART ADJUSTMENTS:** Given the need, your perspective, the facts, and your targeted actions, keep your eyes open and make any changes necessary to stay on target.

Using the *five simple secrets*, you can take charge of any issue in which you want to make change (and in which it is within your power to make change). It is a fantastic formula for self-improvement. For the past 20 years, I've used this technique to place any challenge I come up against into perspective and then use it to take charge of the situation. And it works.

HOW TO USE THE *PRIME* SYSTEM

Having identified both an effective change strategy—the *five simple secrets*—as well as the whole-body approach—the *three key focus areas*—I want now to blend them into a coherent system that will help you take efficient charge of putting your grown-up health and fitness plans totally on-track.

The bulk of the remainder of *Prime* is divided into *three parts*. Each one will revolve completely around one of the *three key focus areas*. For example, the next major section of this book will pertain to developing a MOTIVATED MIND. The information, insights, and strategies in this section will all be delivered in the context of each one of the *five simple secrets*.

I want to strongly emphasize once again that the information that follows is all interactive, with each part of the system having a strong influence on the others. It's impossible to separate the MOTIVATED MIND, for example, from the other *two key focus areas*. To achieve maximum results from your efforts, give equal emphasis to each of the *three key focus areas*.

WHAT ABOUT APPEARANCE?

Following these three parts, there is an additional section dedicated to going several steps beyond the *three key focus areas* and finding ways to look and feel your best. That section is called GREAT LOOKS, and it will target additional aspects of my simple, straightforward philosophies for living life to its fullest.

PART TWO

PRIME
MOTIVATED MIND

The ancestor of every action is a thought.
—RALPH WALDO EMERSON

MY STORY

I had a difficult time writing this book. For the past decade, I've made a significant portion of my living as a writer—so putting words on paper wasn't the issue. My difficulty was in embracing the subject matter that I was going to be writing about. I must confess that, even after selling a proposal for a book about fitness for men over 40, I suddenly found myself less than motivated to write it. The reason was simple: I didn't want to face what was outside my control, which was that my own body was changing with age. To write the book, I knew that I would need to fully accept that inevitable line in the sand that we all face: Growing older.

I realized that I was going to need to make some change in my own life. My feeling was that if I'm going to write a book like this one, I should be living its principles. I should never be handing out advice that I'm not willing to follow myself.

Given that I'd left my most athletic years behind in my mid-30s and had grown relatively sedentary and certainly unmotivated toward fitness, I knew that I was going to have to put myself through some significant changes. It was the only way to get myself into the book, and, by extension, into my own fitness evolution—the same evolution that you may now be facing. If I was going to make a transformation, it had to start with my head.

FIRST CHANGE YOUR MIND

Your physical fitness is directly connected with what happens in your head. Every action you take in life begins in your mind; in your imagination. There is no way around this rule. Before your arm ever lifts a dumbbell, your mind has decided on that action. It has dictated whether your emotions toward what you were preparing to do were positive or negative; your thoughts determined how motivated or complacent you'd be; then—and only then—did your body kick into action.

To change anything about your body, you must first change your mind.

It's impossible to make long-term improvement in your health and well-being without changing the way you think: the way you feel about yourself, and beyond that, how you relate to and act upon those thoughts.

This is one of the greatest tasks facing many 40+ men: an abiding sense of complacency toward fitness and self-image because of long-standing habits of thought and belief. This complacency is then combined with an inaccurate mental picture of what it means to be fit, healthy, and motivated once a man has reached a certain age. We know that, these days, turning 40 isn't necessarily an indication of anything more profound than having a birthday; it certainly doesn't mean an automatic decline into old age. Yet it seems as if our general approach to fitness hasn't quite caught up to this understanding. The way we understand something is influenced by our beliefs, and our beliefs begin—and take hold—in our heads.

Given that, it is of vital importance to begin a balanced *Prime* program with the mind—and by the mind I mean not just simple, everyday thought patterns, but also a man's sense of higher self, his beliefs, and his larger world view. How a man views his world will generally dictate the sort of care he takes of himself. This is a complex matter that will require a man to sit down and focus in on his life very honestly, but it will be along this road that lifelong healthy habits are formed and long-standing poor habits are cast aside.

Your MOTIVATED MIND has many aspects. I break the key areas of concentration down into seven sections. To fully develop a MOTIVATED MIND, you should:

Build self-regard

Write it down

Set goals

Calm yourself

See it happen

Affirm it

Stay consistent

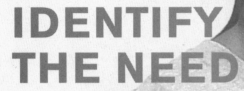

IDENTIFY
THE NEED

Below are some examples of challenges that the grown-up man may face in each of the various areas of concentration. Each is a hurdle that can prevent him from achieving his dreams.

While reading them, see if you can identify with or imagine yourself facing similar hurdles in your own life. Please also bear in mind that these examples may initially seem rather negative. That's because when you want to create change, it's essential to first identify the "negative" quality that you want to move away from, and then to develop a strategy for heading toward the opposite of that quality. So, rather than seeing these examples as negative, please consider using this section to put your finger on a potential need in your own life.

After all, it's very difficult—in fact nearly impossible—to take charge of change if you cannot specifically describe what it is that needs attention. You must name it to claim it.

Here are a few examples of challenges that might stand between a 40+ man and a MOTIVATED MIND:

- A man feels as if his most productive years have slipped away.

- He begins to view himself as "over the hill."

- His lack of self-esteem causes a negative spiral of complacency, inaction, and unhealthy habits.

- He floats aimlessly from day to day, without any concrete plan.

- He cannot tell you where he wants to be next week or next year.

- He clings to goals—be they vague or concrete—set perhaps 20 years earlier and no longer serving their original need.

- He starts projects with great enthusiasm that quickly fades.

- He cannot find ways to fit his healthy lifestyle plans into a hectic life.

- He gives up completely, feeling defeated, when unable to stick with a routine.

- He is frequently stressed and angry at the world around him.

- It feels unfair to him that he is aging and that the advantages of youth have slipped away.

- He can't relax, even in situations that used to make him happy.

- He imagines the worst possible outcome of a given situation.

- He feels cynical about trying to turn his imagination to a positive direction.

- He stops himself from imagining that he could achieve or exceed his secret wildest dreams at this stage of his life.

- He can't track his progress or remember what he did last week, month or year.

- He finds himself repeating some of the same mistakes again and again.

- He has a constant negative loop of conversation—with others and/or inside his head.

- He can tell you all the reasons why things stink, but few reasons why they're good.

- He is unable to honestly come up with anything good to say about himself or his life.

Can you see any part of yourself in these examples? How about slight or broad variations on theme? If so, please understand that we're headed toward solutions. But first, I'd like you to play a game of 20 questions with yourself. This will help you get to know yourself and where you stand on these issues.

Please answer the questions when you have the time, energy, and focus to do a thorough job, and remember that answering honestly and openly will help you move forward. You owe it to yourself to dig deep and open up.

And please do yourself a big favor: Write your answers down. The perspective that you have now won't be the same in a day, a week, or a month—and part of the point of this next exercise is to establish your current perspective.

The order of the steps that I'm recommending in these sections isn't accidental. For example, I'm purposely asking you these questions about your own beliefs and experiences before I tell you about my own philosophies on these subjects, because if I gave you my take on these things (which I'll do in the **Gather the Facts** section), your answers might be influenced by what you'd read. I want your answers to be from your own perspective—and then we'll move on to the facts as I know them.

This next exercise is an important part of getting the maximum benefit from this program.

ESTABLISH YOUR PERSPECTIVE

You are the authority in your own life, not I.
—GARY ZUKAV

Remember that the only "right" answers to the following 20 questions are the perspective that you gain into your own unique situation. This isn't a test; it's an exercise in developing enlightened insight.

QUESTION 1: At this moment in time, are you happy with how you see yourself?

QUESTION 2: What are you capable of doing today to improve the way you see yourself?

QUESTION 3: If you had to honestly rate your motivation for getting into better physical shape and improving your life on a scale of 1 to 10, what number would you give it?

QUESTION 4: How do you feel about your fitness level and habits right now?

QUESTION 5: What do you believe that you need to do to improve this in any way?

QUESTION 6: What are the things that you say (or think) to yourself about the various elements of staying fit and being motivated?

QUESTION 7: Pertaining to #6, would you consider these things more positive or negative?

QUESTION 8: Under general circumstances, do you consider yourself an optimist or a pessimist?

QUESTION 9: Pertaining to #8, how does that influence the way that you see the world?

QUESTION 10: Do you tend to put things off until tomorrow—no matter how important they are—or do you jump right in and do something right away?

QUESTION 11: Under general circumstances, are you a calm person?

QUESTION 12: How do you generally react to the ordinary stresses of life?

QUESTION 13: Do you consider the opinions that others hold of you to be more important than the ones that you hold of yourself?

QUESTION 14: Do you treat your body with respect?

QUESTION 15: How willing are you to change what you decide needs changing?

QUESTION 16: Do you feel helpless against your advancing age?

QUESTION 17: Have you ever stopped yourself from trying something new?

QUESTION 18: What do you consider to be your largest obstacle in life?

QUESTION 19: Is it within your power to overcome this obstacle?

QUESTION 20: What would your life be like—for the next day, month, or year—if you really went after your dreams?

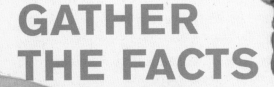

GATHER
THE FACTS

BUILD SELF-REGARD

Many younger men tend to think of a term such as *self-regard* (or the nearly identical, interchangeable *self-esteem*) as one of those touchy-feely, vaguely feminine concepts that should be ignored or avoided. This is where the maturing process can work in a man's favor. Once he gets past his 30s, he generally tends to soften in his view of the world; his warrior's outlook may mellow (as it truly should if he doesn't want to keel over from some stress-related illness). From this softening point of view, a maturing man may well be able to see that how he thinks of himself dictates the level of care he provides for himself—and then, by extension, how well he's able to provide for those who depend on him.

Some people mistake a concept like self-regard for conceit, vanity, or self-centeredness. Actually, a man's true, healthy self-regard is the exact opposite of conceit, which is a condition based upon insecurity. Conceitedness is a false proclamation of greatness, strength, or intelligence that tries desperately to hide some level of insecurity and/or self-loathing. The conceited man is generally, under the surface, the most insecure guy in the room. That's not what we're talking about here. We're talking about a man truly learning to respect himself—his flaws as well as his strengths. A man who takes care of his health and fitness is not vain; his actions are the opposite of vanity; they are acts of self-respect.

A man who truly holds himself in high regard understands that he is valuable and worthy of his own respect. He doesn't need to shout that from the rooftops, he just wears it—comfortably. He also learns to care for himself, just as he would care for someone else whom he held in high regard. He knows that he wouldn't treat anyone badly whom he truly respected; he learns with time and experience that he's just as worthy of the same treatment from himself.

A man who wants to develop truly high self-regard looks inside himself for deeper understanding. He also gathers lessons from his life. The greatest lesson I know about healthy self-esteem is that it is never cast in stone or frozen in time. Everything is constantly shifting in life, and tests are constantly coming our way; inevitable ones such as how we'll handle the aging process. The development of high self-regard occurs when a maturing man learns to integrate the shifting landscape of his life and still make choices and decisions that earn his own respect.

A man who holds himself in high regard learns the difference between bragging that he's the greatest and truly respecting himself and others.

WRITE IT DOWN

OK, so I've already asked you to write out your answers to several personal-analysis questions. By doing this (and if you didn't do it, go back now and answer those questions—they're going to get you on track!) you've already set into motion one of the most valuable tools for creating sustained change: the journal.

I've been keeping extensive journals since I was a teenager. I kept journals of my training and nutrition throughout my competitive career, and I've kept them for my personal life, recording everything from daily events to my own answers to the questions I'll pose in this book—and for many other reasons.

My journals have been like a computer storehouse: a fairly complete record of my life's experience. I can go back several years and tell you what I had for lunch on Tuesday in the third week of November; I can tell you what exercises I did, how I slept, and many other details of my life on any given day.

Through my journals, I've learned what works and what doesn't—not just for my own goals, but also in a larger way. Much of the information I'm sharing in this book had its origins in my journals.

Does it sound like a hassle to you, this journal-keeping business? Well, it shouldn't. There's a key reason why keeping a journal (especially of exercise, nutrition, and general motivation) is so important to the 40+ man: It keeps him from wasting valuable time. It helps him get total efficiency from his efforts.

Keeping a journal helps you live your life consciously, which is essential for taking charge of change and transformation. You'll be able to review where you've been and then set a course for the future. It's an investment in your own well-being. If you're able to learn from where you've been, not only by paying attention but also by making a permanent record, you can do what you've set out to do with greater clarity and efficiency. As a 40+ man fighting the tide of aging (and perhaps only getting on track after many years off), efficiency is vitally important—not just for your waistline, but for your health. The faster and more efficiently you turn your fitness life around, the faster you will realize the health benefits associated with balanced and well-planned self-care.

It may seem like a hassle at first, but months or years from now, as you read where you've been (perhaps smiling at your rapid progress), you'll be mighty proud that you took the time to write it all down.

SET GOALS

You're always setting goals in life. Whether you do so consciously or not is up to you, but where you are in your fitness life is a complete reflection of how you've set your goals: how accurately you've set them and how effectively you've acted on them.

If a 40+ man wants the second half of his life to be high-quality, he has no time to waste while getting himself healthy and fit. The way to optimize the time is to learn to take charge of the goal-setting process.

Every good self-improvement program depends on short-and long-term goals. My approach is to always focus on what I want to achieve today, this week, this month, this year, and so forth. And I write it all down. In other words, it isn't enough to simply say "I want this, this, and this." The act of writing it down roots your goal in reality, and you'll then find ways to act on what you have imagined for yourself—today, tomorrow, and onward into the future.

Many men feel that it is enough to simply say that they'll work out more and eat better; that literally writing out goals is a waste of time. I'm here to tell you that it isn't. First of all, how do you really know where you want to go and what you want to achieve if you don't give it strong thought? Beyond that, how are you supposed to remember exactly what it is you're aiming for if you don't have written record of your goals?

Efficiency is the term I keep returning to in all of this motivational work. Your efforts on your own behalf should be all about discovering the most efficient ways of getting from Point A to Point B. Setting yourself up with clear, written goals is the fastest, most efficient way to get what you truly want from your efforts.

I'm hard on the idea of quick-fix solutions because I truly feel that while they seem to solve a problem over the short term, in the long run they leave you worse off than you were at the beginning. Let me say from experience that writing down your goals is just about the most effective and real quick-fix there is. The fastest way to get what you desire is to know—concretely—where you're headed.

CALM YOURSELF

We live in a world filled with stress. Any man over 40 already knows that. In order to become fully fit and healthy, you must find ways to lessen the stress load.

As men, we are often given images of what it means to be motivated. Often these images are very "rah-rah," high-adrenaline, jump-up-and-down physical demonstrations. The problem is that this sort of over-the-top enthusiasm can't really be maintained over the long term. And adding this sort of stress into a 40+ life will likely cause more health problems than it will solve. That's why I encourage a calmer, more centered approach to staying on-target. In my experience, the guy who yells and screams his way through his workout isn't motivating himself, he's trying to attract attention. You'll want to take a more mature approach than that.

Think of the difference between some over-adrenalized linebacker in a pregame locker room, screaming, banging his head against things. How healthy would that technique be in your everyday life? Now think of the centered calmness of a professional golfer finessing his way toward his goal—focusing, concentrating, breathing, staying in control. I want you to see your efforts more in this light. It's far healthier for you as a mature man to create change through a centered, focused effort; after all, you aren't trying to scare an enemy into submission here; you're trying to take yourself toward an embrace of a good healthy life. Getting yourself to relax is an important step toward doing that. Calming your mind leads you away from stress and toward the ability to see things as they truly are. Think about the difference between how clearly you see something when you're blind with rage and the way you would see the same thing if your emotions were more calm. The same concept applies to your efforts here.

I think that because so many images about exercise depict men grunting and screaming their way through workouts, and because so many men believe that training is purely a grunt-and-groan activity, there is a general misunderstanding of how to find a truly focused path in fitness.

Returning again to the idea that as a 40+ man you need efficient methods for achieving long-term success, I encourage you to approach your physical exercise as more of a meditative, focus-oriented activity. Shifting toward a calmer approach to training (and to life) helps a man hold the ravages of stress-induced illness to a minimum and helps his life go smoother along the way.

Let's be frank: stress kills, and it also makes you age poorly along the way. I want you to start practicing techniques that will calm your mind and spirit; that will help you find a centered peacefulness in your life.

When you're outside the gym, I encourage you to build your motivation not by bouncing off the walls, but rather through relaxing your mind and beginning to understand the power of inner quiet.

SEE IT HAPPEN

To create positive change, you should have a firm picture in your mind of what you want. As I've said, everything that becomes an action begins in your imagination. So, before you embark on any program of change, I would encourage you to develop your skills of assertive visualization, which is a proactive method of blending mental relaxation techniques with a purposeful guidance of the images that you see in your mind about a particular subject.

Assertive visualization is the process of taking control of the mental images that you see about any particular subject. On the other hand, passive visualization is the process of simply allowing whatever passes through your mind—be it a positive or negative contribution to your life—simply unfold without doing anything to alter its direction. Assertive visualization is simply taking charge of the movie in your head and changing it to one that more accurately serves your true needs.

I've used my own form of visualization for decades in conjunction with my training. Before other athletes learned the power of creating their own positive mental movies, people used to make fun of me. That's OK; I know that taking control of my own mind made me a more successful athlete.

There were three key times when I felt that assertive visualization worked best:

- Just before and just after a workout;

- At the beginning and the end of the day;

- During exercise.

By taking control of the movie that plays in your head, you'll connect more directly with your body and experience far greater results, because your mind is an incredibly powerful thing. It will create for you what you imagine—within reason—about your circumstances. I'm not saying that all you need to do is imagine often enough that you are in amazing shape and—presto!—you'll suddenly be in great shape. You still must do the work. But think about it: You always put more effort into something that you have positive feelings about. You begin having positive feelings about something by way of how you imagine it. Your imagination is most receptive to positive, assertive guidance when you're in a very relaxed state. You can change your fitness life simply by beginning to see a different picture of yourself. That picture will help you take better care of your body, which will lead you to feel better about yourself. Can you see how this upward loop can be the fastest way to turn your fitness life around?

AFFIRM IT

In addition to using assertive visualization to fine-tune how you see things unfolding, you should also examine the things that you say to yourself. Does your language (out loud and in your mind) about the various aspects of your fitness life reflect a positive outlook, or a negative one? In other words, do you say things to yourself that are uplifting, or down-dragging? Your visual imagination is powerful, and so are the things that you say to yourself.

What you tell yourself directly influences the outcome of what you desire. Your internal (and external) language will set you up for success or failure.

Do you have a project that you're excited about—one that gets you up out of bed in the morning and keeps you up late at night? Think about the things you say to yourself when you're working at this thing that you're so passionate about. Now imagine a project that you dread—that you'd avoid at all costs. What kinds of things do you say to yourself about this? Probably that it's boring, or stupid, or whatever negative thing you can think of. What do you think the outcome of those negative words is going to be? Most likely, it will make the project what you say it is. You may not believe that your words are that powerful, but they are.

Without trying to sound too "Pollyanna" about this: The things you say to yourself about something will—with enough energy—make your belief true. Say over and over to yourself enough times that you're an over-the-hill-fat-no-muscle-stroke-waiting-to-happen, and in some form or another you'll become that. The manifestation may be physical, or it may only be a negative affect on your overall self-image, which will then make you take poor care of yourself (because, well, why bother?), but one way or another, your words will become a reality. Your efforts will be a direct reflection of your verbal belief system. To very loosely paraphrase an old saying: If you can't say anything nice to yourself, then learn how to change until you can. Your health and the quality of your life may depend on learning to talk to yourself in more positive ways.

STAY CONSISTENT

When a man begins an exercise program, he sometimes has a hard time imagining that his efforts are paying off. It's difficult to look ahead and see how today's workout will equal gains that may not show themselves for several weeks. This is where many men hurt their efforts. When they don't see instant results, they give up. Consistency is the only way through this dilemma. Your outlook and your actions must continue on a steady course; in your imagination you must be able to see (visualize) that if you put in one day after another, your efforts will pay off.

Consistent action is the bridge between the goals that you set and your achievement of them. Consistent action taken toward a desired goal is what separates fantasy from accomplishment. Anyone can talk about getting in better shape, but eventually the rubber has to meet the road. Be a man of action, but don't simply take action today; take it tomorrow and the day after and the day after that—until you have achieved your dreams. Relax your mind. See this clearly. Tell yourself it is possible. Go out and do it.

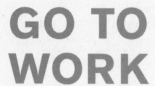

GO TO WORK

Here are the basic steps for putting the important elements of your MOTIVATED MIND into action:

BUILD SELF-REGARD

1. Learn how to distinguish between temporary, quick-fix fitness ideals (losing 20 pounds in ten days, no matter how unhealthy the method) and those that are longer lasting (learning how to be consistent in your efforts for six months or a year). Really examine how your long-term self-respect will benefit from taking a gentler, more caring route to getting healthy and fit. (And here's a hint: There's never anything healthy or esteem-building about crash diets, as I'll discuss in an upcoming chapter.)

2. Consciously learn to ask yourself: Is this action going to contribute to my well-being or subtract from it?

3. Learn how to truly differentiate between those aspects of your physical body and emotional makeup that are within your power to change and those that are not. Don't underestimate the important power of this step. It can mean the difference between a life of bitterness (with the accompanying belief that progress is beyond your grasp) and the uplifting enlightenment of knowing where to put your best-directed physical efforts toward realistic improvements. It will also illuminate the places where you should simply work harder toward greater self-acceptance.

4. Balance an acceptance of your perceived weaknesses (for example, some aspect of your physical body or appearance that you see as flawed) with your desire for positive change. Understand that true self-esteem grows from acceptance of our full selves. When you learn how to differentiate between aspects of yourself that can be changed (things like body-fat level and muscle tone, for example) and those that cannot (like basic bone structure and chronological age) you can get to the heart of liking yourself for who you are.

5. Sit in a quiet, private place with a pad of paper and a pen. Close your eyes and take ten deep, relaxing breaths. Now open your eyes, pick up the pen, and without thinking begin to write down all the things you don't like about yourself. Keep writing until you run out of steam (or until five minutes pass). Now close your eyes again, take ten deep, relaxing breaths, open your eyes, and without thinking begin to write down everything that you like about yourself. Write until you run out of steam. Now compare the lists in a detached manner. How many of the things on the "don't like" list are out of your control to change? How many on the "like" list are?

6. Using the above writing, separate your lists into those things that you can reasonably expect to change (once again, look to things like body fat, muscle tone, outlook, diet, and so forth). Now examine this list of aspects that are actually changeable, and separate out the ones that you have the time and energy to concentrate on trying to improve. You've just taken an important step toward setting some raw priorities.

7. Every morning when you get out of bed and every night before falling asleep, take a few minutes to focus on some aspect of yourself that you truly respect.

This may initially sound pretty touchy-feely, but ask yourself this: Do you want to get better? Isn't all that concern about what's touchy-feely really just worry about what someone else will think? Do you really, truly care what anyone else thinks about your efforts to put your health and fitness on track? Either way, realize that this is a silent, in-the-head exercise; nobody's going to know you're doing it but you. And it will help you improve. Do you follow my drift here?

8. Understand that true self-regard isn't about superficial changes. You can get big muscles or lose all your fat, but if you don't work on your outlook and go inside yourself and dig deeper into the way you regard yourself, you won't really have changed as deeply as you could have. In other words, don't just lift the weights; dig deep, be introspective, and lift your spirits.

9. Stop measuring yourself against unreasonable standards. When you're past 40, your body may or may not (based on a combination of your genetics and how much work you put in) look like that of a 25-year-old fitness-magazine cover model. So what? Embrace who you are right now. In upcoming chapters, I'm going to show you how to make yourself look as young as you can—according to how much effort you want to put in—but go beyond that. Work toward an embrace of your age, your condition, and your circumstances. Get off your own back if you don't look like a supermodel. Measuring yourself against that standard will never do you an ounce of good and will only take you further away from improving on who you really are.

10. Set aside any cynicism that you've built up over the years. Learn to open your heart up again to the possibilities in life. Yes, we've all had hard knocks; yes, we've all been screwed over somewhere along the line. That's life. But don't let that outlook shut you away from believing that a little bit (or a lot) of magic can't happen in your own life. It'll be through that re-embrace of a childlike (but not immature and childish) sense of possibility, combined with your mature work ethic, that you'll be able to take major steps in your own wellness evolution.

WRITE IT DOWN

1. Begin today. Get yourself a notebook of some sort (or open a computer folder—although in general I recommend a paper notebook because of porta-

bility) and dedicate it to this cause. Don't delay. Don't get caught up in waiting until you have just the right kind of paper—that's nothing but a stall tactic.

2.   Start by answering with complete honesty all of the "Establish Your Perspective" questions in each of the five sections of this book. Date the top of the page so that you can know the day that you began to change your life.

3.   Set aside at least five quiet, private minutes every day to record your workouts (including such things as exercises, repetitions, weights, duration, energy, and feelings) and what you eat; record the amount of sleep you got, its quality, what time you got up, and what time you went to bed; write down how dedicated (or unmotivated) you were in your fitness efforts. Dedicate at least one full page to this record.

4.   Keep doing this every day. It is said that it takes at least three consistent weeks to establish any new habit. Dedicate—promise yourself and keep your word— at least three solid weeks to making this valuable habit take hold.

5.   On a daily basis, dedicate at least one additional page (I actually do three each day) to a frank dialogue with yourself about your life. Make it a completely free-flowing, stream-of-consciousness effort. Don't worry about grammar, spelling, sentence structure, or logic. It's best to do this first thing in the morning, just out of bed, before the world has descended on your life. It has little to do with your fitness life, but it is a direct link to how you're feeling about yourself and your place in the world—and that is at least tangentially linked to your overall health and well-being.

6.   Be absolutely, rock-solid honest in your journal. It does you no good to exaggerate, make up workouts, skip over days when your diet wasn't good, and so forth. If you miss a day at the gym, write it down; use the journal to figure out why. (Were you tired? Stressed? Lazy? Overtrained?) If you break your nutrition program, write it down. You've got to use the journal properly to get the full benefit, and the only way to do that is to be raw and honest.

7.   With this level of honesty, it is essential to keep your journal totally to yourself. Don't show it to anyone. The last thing you need is your (fill-in-the-blank) analyzing, critiquing, scrutinizing your honest feelings and the record of your efforts. You are also far more likely to be completely honest if you know that no one else will read what you've written.

8.   If you skip a day of journaling, pick right back up again. Consider doing an overview of any skipped days (it is perhaps telling that most people I know skip

journaling on days they've gone off a nutrition plan or strayed from other healthy habits). But write an overview: Did you train? How? What did you eat? Things like that.

9. Do not, under any circumstances, think that you must be a good writer to keep a journal. Your use of language is relevant only to you. You only have to write so that you understand it. Begin with the basics and, who knows, perhaps you'll discover that you love to write things down. I've seen it happen.

10. Realize that journaling is an exercise in conscious living, and that in general it is far easier to simply glide along in life without examining or reviewing our actions or feelings. This sort of hands-off living, combined with the natural changes in the 40+ body, will not lead you to the healthy outcome that you desire. Take a few minutes each day to make this investment in yourself.

SET GOALS

1. Start with your journal right in front of you. You must write out what you want, so begin a section for your goals. Any goals that you set for yourself should be stated in the positive—in ways that you find motivating.

2. Only begin a goal-setting session when you have the time to give it your full attention. Find a relaxed, quiet place, sit down, and allow yourself plenty of time to do this right.

3. Understand that the goals you set for yourself must be rooted in reality. They must take into consideration your own body, your own work ethic, your own willingness to invest time and effort. If you don't begin with reality and instead simply—wildly—project out desires that have nothing to do with what is under your control to change, you only set yourself up for massive disappointment which will likely lead to giving up.

4. Be willing to reach beyond where you are now. While understanding what is real and achievable, don't underestimate what you are actually capable of achieving. Just because you've never been there before doesn't mean that the journey is impossible.

5. Understand that while keeping your goals rooted in reality and your potential to reach beyond where you are now, you should also take into account your own history of follow-through on new ideas. It is all well and good to sit down and tell yourself that you'll change your diet and do such and such exercises this

many times each week, but finding a means of following through is a big step beyond that. If procrastination is an issue that you face, consider making it your number-one goal to overcome that trait. Decide that you will put off procrastinating. Make your wellness evolution so important that you can't imagine not avoiding the efforts directed toward your top priorities—your goals.

6. In your journal, write out your honest answers to the following questions about your fitness quest:

    What do you want to achieve by next week?

    Next month?

    Next year?

    Where do you see yourself in five years?

    What can you do now to start that off on the right foot?

7. When writing out your honest goals for your personal fitness evolution, concentrate on:

    ■ Physical body

    Short-term (today through one year)

    Long-term (one year and beyond)

    ■ Nutrition

    Short-term

    Long-term

    ■ Personal development

    Short-term

    Long-term

    ■ Personal perceptions

    Short-term

    Long-term

8. Now sit in a quiet place with your journal. Breathe yourself into a state of relaxation and close your eyes. Imagine each area in which you are creating goals. Imagine the changes that you want to make. Now open your eyes and, in the categories listed in #7 above, begin to write out your goals.

9. In setting your goals, it's as essential that you find something powerful to go *toward* as it is to identify conditions that you want to go *away from*. In other

words, if one of your fitness goals is to lose 10 pounds, you're going away from something—the fat. To make the goal truly effective and efficient, you must establish something equally compelling to go toward—perhaps building greater muscle tone and flexibility. Here's a nutritional example: If you're going away from a diet heavy in junk food, you should make it an equal goal to go toward eating totally healthy foods.

10. After you have written out your goals, make a contract with yourself. Use the goals that you've set; write them out in a clear, concise way so that there's no question about what you want to achieve, and then put some language along the bottom of the page that says something along the lines of: *I [your name] promise to myself that I will do everything within my power to fulfill these goals. I understand that I am working in my own best interests and that by fulfilling this obligation I am improving my health and my life.* Then sign it. You have just entered into an important contract with yourself. Honor it as you would a contract with anyone else. You deserve it.

11. Once each week, turn to the goal section of your journal and conduct a personal review. Look at how you've been doing compared to what you contracted to do. Weigh for yourself, in a totally honest way, whether or not the places where your efforts and your goals turned out to be different were in fact improvements or places where you need to try harder. Sometimes the goals we set will need adjustment according to new realities in our lives. Be willing to adjust, but don't do it only to let yourself off the hook.

CALM YOURSELF

1. Learning to control your breathing is the first essential step in any effective relaxation exercise. Most men breathe in a very shallow way, and this tends to add tension to the body and the mind. Begin right now by breathing in through your nose until your lungs are completely full. As you breathe in, consciously seek out any tight places in your body (perhaps your neck and shoulder blades). As your lungs fill, purposely relax one tension area a little bit. Now allow yourself to exhale—slowly and under relaxed control. Consciously relax another physical-tension spot. Repeat this deep breathing at least 10 times. Your mind may scream with impatience. Let it. It is hooked on tension. Ignore it and relax. Breathe deeply and allow the tension to be released from your body.

2. As you repeat these deep breaths, pay attention. Don't simply focus on the tight places in your body; also be attentive to the places in your head that rebel

against this process of slowing down. Find a deeper level of peace with each breath. Practice this deep-breathing technique first thing in the morning and at the end of your day. Do it until it becomes fairly simple.

3. After practicing paying attention to your breath (and this practice isn't competitive, so it may take you a few minutes or a week to feel as if you're getting it) I'd like you to try a deeper level of relaxation; more of a meditation. Now, a lot of men are pretty cynical about the notion of meditating. It sounds to them like some sort of vaguely unmasculine, new-agey, woo-woo thing. If you're one of those men, I'm asking you to set that aside for the moment and just try something new. You may be amazed at how much better you feel. There is nothing unmasculine about learning to take control of your body, and that's all meditation is—a technique for taking charge of your body's relaxation response. Now, sit or lie in a comfortable place. Make sure that you'll have at least 15 quiet, uninterrupted minutes. Close your eyes. Relax them. Start taking your deep breaths, and pay attention to your tension spots. With each breath, release a bit more tension. You can further direct this by beginning at your feet—relaxing them—and then moving up your legs, torso, arms, and so forth, each step along the way relaxing every body part until you've gotten to the top of your head. Breathe deep and steady.

4. If your mind wanders during this exercise, let it. The idea isn't that you'll go into some sort of mystical trance. Chances are good that your thoughts won't just stop coming, but with time they will slow down. So when your mind throws things at you, don't react. Instead, just sort of look at it—in a detached unemotional way—and simply let it drift past. You may be amazed at how this happens. Every time you do it—just let an interfering thought simply drift in and out—you take greater charge of yourself. Tension and stress don't necessarily come from the events in our lives, but rather from our reactions to them. You've just taken Step One in learning to overcome stress, and it probably wasn't even that hard.

5. When you are in this quiet place, after you've relaxed your way through all your body parts, just hang out there. The television, or the telephone, or whatever, will still be around after you finish. Spend some time just hanging out inside your own head. You may be amazed to discover how noisy the world you live in truly is, once you've found a quiet place inside yourself. When you have finished—after five minutes, or twenty—allow yourself to come back slowly. Come back into the world the same way that you relaxed your way out of it. (It

might also be helpful to use one of the Flexibility Sequences from the FIT BODY section to reinvigorate your body and literally stretch out your relaxation time.)

6. Once you've begun to use this simple technique, you can start to use it in a wide variety of circumstances. With practice, you can usually trigger your relaxation mechanism within five or six deep, focused breaths. Imagine that you're stuck in traffic or in some long-winded meeting, or that you're encountering another of the daily stressors of modern life. See yourself in one of those situations—it's usually a sense of having no control that drives us into a stressed-out rage, right? So instead of allowing the situation to control you, turn it on its head. Take control of your response by consciously acknowledging your building stress and beginning the deep, tension-releasing breaths. After about 10 of them, your reaction to the situation will probably be much calmer, far more within your control. You won't change the traffic, but you will change your response to it. And that will make you a healthier man.

7. I like to use my deep-breathing meditation before workouts. Many men believe that workouts should be about gut-wrenching, grunt-and-groan efforts. As you'll read in future sections, I take a very different view. Your workouts should be an opportunity to tune your attention skills; they should be focused, because that will exponentially increase their efficiency. I like to do a short version of my meditation (perhaps five minutes) before I go into the gym or out for a run. It helps pull my attention inward, relaxing my mind, allowing me to focus in on whatever parts of my body are about to be worked. I also see this as a key time to blend in my assertive visualization exercises, and I'll probably add several important affirmations. Doing this helps turn my workout into an extended, active type of meditation.

SEE IT HAPPEN

1. If you think that you are unable to visualize, please understand that this is a skill that can be improved with practice. You don't have to have a big Technicolor movie unfold before your eyes to visualize effectively. You are more accurately trying to build a visual sense in your mind. You already do it in one way or another. If you daydream about something that happened in your past, you're visualizing. So, it may help to think of this as directed daydreaming. The first step is to get a concrete sense of what it feels like. Look at an object in front of

you (it can be anything), and examine it carefully. Now close your eyes and sense that object—see it, or feel it, or do whatever it is that you do in your mind to duplicate the sensation of it. That's visualization.

2. The greatest fitness use for assertive visualization is imagining how you will look and feel as a result of your directed efforts. It's a way of invigorating your goals—turning them into positive actions—by seeing your outcomes in advance. The best way to do this is to use your meditation breathing technique to bring yourself into a relaxed and focused state. Then create a picture of yourself as you want to look and feel in, say, 10 weeks, if you were to put your best effort toward your goals. Make the image you have of yourself absolutely real; get a sense of place by seeing yourself in an active way—perhaps running or out on the town looking amazing, fit and glowing. Hold this moving image before your eyes. Allow it to fuel your desire for change.

3. When doing the exercise above, it is essential to use yourself in your visualization. An old technique for getting a better body is to cut out a picture of your own head, then find a picture of the body that you dream of having and cut that out, and then put your head on that other person's body, imagining with all your power that it is you. I strongly discourage this technique. It says that your body isn't good enough. Rather than being a sound motivation technique, it sets you up for failure. First of all, many men who use this technique tend to select pictures of bodies far more developed than they themselves have the time or energy to become. Second, what does it say about your self-perception that you would trade your body for someone else's. Instead, get a strong image in your mind of *your* body, your bone structure, your muscle shapes. Imagine all of those unique aspects of yourself taken to their maximum level. *Visualize yourself at your best.*

4. I also like to use visualization prior to my workouts. Along with relaxation techniques, it is a powerful way to get myself focused on what I'm about to do. This is a technique that elite athletes have begun to use with a great deal of success. It builds the sort of genuine motivation that I described earlier as being so diametrically opposed to the "head-banging, screaming and yelling" techniques that so many men mistakenly believe are the keys to athletic performance. No matter what activity you're preparing for, run a detailed tape of it in your mind. If you are doing a weight workout, spend a few relaxed minutes in your parked car (if you drove to the gym) imagining—seeing—the exercises that you'll do. See yourself doing them perfectly, with excellent form (a concept that I'll discuss at length later) and great intensity. Allow your imaginary workout to exceed your own usual performance—by a bit. Don't make it unrealistic. Your

mind won't buy it. If you usually do your barbell curls with 60 pounds, use that in your visualization; just make it all perfect—form, environment, focus, feeling. You can "see" your way to the best workouts of your life by keying yourself before you ever step into the training environment.

5. You can continue this technique while doing the actual exercise. This is an especially valuable practice to use with exercises that require focused energy, such as weight training. Now, this is an area in which I take a slightly different position than many others do. I don't see my time in the gym as a "social hour." I don't think that you should carry on a conversation while you're doing your sets. Here's an observation from someone who's trained at an elite level for 20 years: The results that you'll get out of your training will be in exact proportion to the focused energy you put in. The men I see who turn the gym into a social hour rarely show any improvement from one month or year to the next. If they focused, it would be a whole different story. In the gym you should be focused enough so that carrying on a conversation seems counterproductive. The most efficient use of your time between sets of exercises is visualizing your next set. While you catch your breath, see the next perfect thing you're going to do. Your training should be an extension of your meditation. This is perhaps one of my greatest secrets for amazing results: Be distracted, and you'll get nowhere. Focus in, see what you want, and you'll achieve your dreams.

6. Don't think that the gym is the only place where this technique is valuable. You can use it while power-walking, stretching, cycling, and on and on. Any activity that you are doing that's directed toward your fitness goal will benefit directly from active and assertive visualization. See what you want. See yourself moving effortlessly, stretching with the amazing flexibility of a gymnast. When you see it in your mind, you create a bridge between your body and the deepest aspects of yourself; you trigger the mechanism that allows you to perform at a level you may have never experienced before. This is one of those lessons that a mature man can learn, and that can give him a distinct advantage over younger men. When we're young, we take so much for granted—performance, recovery, grace, speed, and so on. When you use your imagination, it reinforces the efforts of your body in ways that get you—and will keep you—totally on your fitness track.

AFFIRM IT

1. Create a page in your journal. Every day for one week, listen to the things that you say to yourself about your body, the way you eat, how you feel about your-

self, your appearance. Record it all. Pay special attention to anything negative that you think or say out loud: "I'm so fat," or "I'm getting so saggy," or "What's one more bacon-double-cheeseburger gonna hurt?" Be honest and willing to listen. You might be surprised at how much you're ignoring in your ongoing inner dialogue. The things that you say to yourself create your world—or, at the very least, they create your perception of the world. Your perception of yourself and your world dictates many of your actions, especially ones that could benefit you. So open your ears to that you might be insulting yourself, and then be willing to change.

2.   To affirm something means to make it firm. An affirmation—unlike the negative things that we may think and feel about ourselves—is something positive that you say to yourself and that sets your goals in motion. I create affirmations for myself by looking first at all the negative things I may feel—about my body, my emotions, my accomplishments, and so on—to get an indication of what needs work. If I'm criticising myself about my improvement levels, I'll create an affirmation that's the opposite of my self-criticism. And that is essential: In order for affirmations to work, they must be stated in the reasonable positive. You probably know what I mean by "positive," but what about "reasonable"? Once again, this means that what I am affirming is within my grasp. For example, if I'm down on my accomplishments, it's not reasonable to counter-affirm with something like: "I am the world's greatest astronaut." The statement has no basis in reality. Since I'm a writer it would be better for me to say something like: "Every day, I am becoming a better writer." This is an affirmation rooted in my reality. It reaches for something beyond where I am now. It is stated in a positive and active voice. These are essential ingredients.

3.   Affirmations aren't limited to positive statements. They can also be what I call directed questions. These are questions that I design for my particular circumstances and that I know will lead me to a positive—or affirming—answer. They're questions that can relate to any topic: in the context of your fitness goals, they can address such issues as food, exercise, outlook, motivation, appearance, self-perception. Be careful, though, when you use directed questions. If you're in a cynical mood, or things aren't going very well, it's easy to give yourself some pretty snide answers. All that will do is undermine your efforts. Instead, when you're in those circumstances, use directed questions to turn your mood in a more positive direction.

4.   Affirmations and directed questions can both be used throughout the day. My suggestion is that you use them four or five times each day for the first three

weeks. You do this to build a positive habit that you're conscious of practicing, and then, with enough time, it will evolve into something—like brushing your teeth—that you couldn't imagine not doing at least twice each day.

5.   Use your journal to keep track of how many times each day you go through your affirmations. This is a simple way to stay on top of it until it becomes automatic. Write it down just as you would your workouts or diet.

6.   Get out your journal. On a new page, I want you to create at least 10 positive affirmations for your daily use. You'll also need to get your hands on some index cards. Once you have a final version in your journal, I advise you to write your affirmations out on these cards and carry them with you during the day.

7.   As you create an affirmation, write it in such a way that—as explained above—it's both reasonable and positive, and use simple language indicating that you're already performing this action. For example, if I want to create an affirmation to help me stay on track with my diet, I'll write: "Today I enjoy eating clean, healthy foods. I love the way it makes my body feel young and energetic."

8.   Now in your journal begin to write some affirmations for your own needs. Here are some of my favorites:

For my body:

I love how exercising every day makes my body feel young and energetic.

I'm getting in better and better shape every day.

My exercise focus is unshakable. The focus helps me grow.

I do only that which helps my body grow strong and healthy.

I exercise with perfect form and focus for perfect results.

For my diet:

For this meal, on this day, I eat only that which makes me healthy.

I am committed to the power of my eating plan. It is unshakable.

My hunger is mine to control. I am in charge of my appetite.

I am too important to fill myself with junk food.

For my outlook:

I am grateful for the beauty in my life.

I am thankful for my power and health.

I live today understanding that I have happiness as my destiny.

I am young in mind and spirit.

For my health:

I am flooded with amazing health and energy.

My body is a temple of healing and abundance.

I am youthful, energized, and healthy in every moment.

Today, every step I take contributes to my health.

My body is whole, my mind is calm, my spirit is strong.

9. Now work on some directed questions in your journal. After you have five or six, write each one on an individual index card. Here are a few of my directed questions, some related to fitness, many dedicated to general outlook—which, in case you haven't noticed yet, is directly linked to fitness in my philosophy:

   What do I have to be grateful for in my life?

   How can I make this the most productive day possible?

   How would I feel tonight if I took perfect care of myself today?

   What can I do today to keep myself feeling young?

   How can I accomplish my goals today?

   Are there any areas of my fitness life that I've been neglecting lately?

10. When you've written each affirmation and each directed question on its own index card, use a rubber band to hold your stack of cards together, and carry them with you. Use your cards several times each day. With affirmations, read each statement to yourself and really feel it—as if it is absolutely true. As you go through your cards, try to repeat each affirmation at least 10 times. With the directed questions, use these the very first thing when you get out of bed. Answer the questions honestly, but in a positive manner, and really feel what you are answering. Set any cynicism aside. This stuff works. In order to do something different in your life, you must first change your mind. This is the way to do that.

11. I also use my affirmations after I've meditated. In a completely relaxed state, I'll pull out my cards and run through my positive statements. In addition to that, I'll come up with an affirmation for while I'm working out. In between sets of exercises or during my run, I'll repeat the same affirmation over and over again. As I stated earlier, I see my workouts as a form of focused, moving medita-

tion—exercise not just for my body but also for my mental focus—so using a powerful affirmation is a way to pull myself deeper into my focus. It helps me make my beliefs stronger, and that in turn helps my body to respond faster. My current favorite: I exercise with perfect form and focus for perfect results.

STAY CONSISTENT

1. Take responsibility for getting yourself on track. No one can truly stop you from taking care of yourself but you. If your significant other or your friends aren't supportive of your efforts, don't use that as an excuse not to begin or to quit. See it instead as a challenge. Know that taking care of yourself sometimes makes others feel insecure about the way they treat themselves. See their resistance for what it really is and, instead of letting it stop you, allow it to make you stronger.

2. On the other hand, you should also be aware—especially if you're new to all this fitness stuff—that it's easy to go overboard in expecting everyone around you to be just as enthusiastic as you are about your newfound programs and philosophies. You can convert the willing, but unsolicited preaching generally repels people. Be sure in your actions and beliefs—for yourself. Find consistency not through the agreement of others, but through becoming centered and relaxed with your own choices. If you want to help others to discover the benefits you've found, lead through deeds, not words. Let the actions and outcomes of your new lifestyle and not an unwanted sermon, be the inspiration.

3. There will be times when your mind simply rebels against doing another workout, eating a clean meal, or some other aspect of your program. While the majority of your efforts should be done with full mental attention, focus, and consciousness, there are times when you will simply need to let your body take over. Just going through the motions—as long as it doesn't turn into a longstanding habit—is a good way to get through a minor slump. For example, if your mind is dead-set against doing your exercises, instead of giving in and just skipping them altogether, tell yourself that you're going to do a "half-effort" workout. Go to your training environment (gym, track, whatever) and simply begin a light workout. Tell yourself that this is all you plan to do. Chances are that your body will get warmed up and your mind will become engaged (especially if you use some affirmations), and you may just have a great workout. If your mind doesn't engage, then you'll simply have had a lighter workout, but will still have made progress.

4. On the other hand, if your mind is willing but your body is genuinely fatigued, this could be a signal of something altogether different. You may not be recuperating fully from your previous workouts, or you may be eating too few calories or not getting enough sleep. (These are issues important to the 40+ man, and I'll cover them in later sections.) If this is the case, then your powers of honest observation are going to have to come to your aid. Review your journal and ask yourself if you are truly weary or just being lazy. Relax your head with your deep-breathing exercises, and go inside for the answer. You may be surprised at how much information our own bodies begin to provide us with once we begin to ask ourselves for assistance.

5. Don't look too quickly for amazing results. If you begin a program and expect your body to make overnight changes, you may become disappointed and quit when it doesn't. The sorts of changes that you're trying to make take time and patience. Know that you will need to keep coming in and going at it. Think of your fitness goals as like a savings account where the interest grows and compounds with time. As you exercise, allow your mind to extrapolate the results out beyond the moment. Focus on the present, but also see ahead. Use your imagination to visualize your achieved goals and to spark your desire to do everything within your power to take yourself there.

6. If you miss a workout (or several) or screw up on your diet, don't give up. There is more than one way to measure consistency. Having a perfect "attendance" record is one way. However, we are all human, and life sometimes simply gets in the way. If for any reason you miss workouts or go off-diet, simply begin again. Go back to your journal, record your observations, and then go back on track. Don't beat yourself up; learn from it and go forward.

7. Consider finding a training partner for your workouts. This person should have similar goals and should definitely be on the same wavelength regarding focus during a workout. If you want to make progress, don't start training with the gym chatterbox. As I've already stated, I have yet to see anyone who has a reputation for being a gabber in the gym make any sort of significant gains. The big talkers are usually too busy interrupting other people's efforts. Think of a training partnership as something of a mini-marriage. Your goals must mesh well with your partner's, or no one is going to be happy.

8. Consider hiring a trainer to keep you consistent. Having a trainer helps many men commit to showing up each day and getting the work done. I have one

major caution about the current trend of everybody and his brother hanging out a trainer's shingle: Your trainer must be totally committed to your efforts. While you are exercising, every ounce of your trainer's energy and focus should be on you and your exercise form (more on this later). Your trainer is not supposed to be a great conversationalist (at least not during your workout), and even with supervision, you should still observe the dictates of focus. Your trainer should support this fully. I cannot stress this notion enough: Talking your way through a workout (and being otherwise distracted and unfocused) is a sure way to undermine your goals and minimize your results. A good trainer knows this. A lousy trainer doesn't. He or she should also understand the unique needs of the 40+ body regarding recuperation and injury, and be nearly obsessed with a concept I call exercise perfection (more on this coming up). I've seen men helped by trainers and hurt by them. Interview a potential candidate thoroughly before signing on for any paid sessions.

MAKE SMART ADJUSTMENTS

Working to develop a MOTIVATED MIND through all of the concepts I've discussed is an ongoing process. Even if you achieve your goals today or this week, that doesn't mean you won't need to invest your attention and effort toward them next week or next month. It also doesn't mean that your circumstances won't have changed with time.

Pay attention. This is my primary piece of advice, and one of the most valuable in this entire book. You should be opening yourself up in such a way that you are attentive to what is happening in your life. Many of us live our lives as if we're half-asleep. The road to total fitness and wellness—especially after the easy assumptions of youth are behind us—is entered upon through waking up, understanding what we are doing to ourselves, and making positive changes.

Observe your actions. Use your journal. Ask yourself on a consistent basis if you are on or off track with what you have set out to do.

If you discover through careful reflection that you haven't been consistent, change your approach today. And then stick with it tomorrow. And then the day after that. Don't beat yourself up or use a lapse as an excuse to quit. Refocus and begin again.

Look at how well your goals are serving you each week. Be willing to shift either your approach to them or a goal itself if it needs adjustment. If you are open and you observe your progress (or lack of it), you'll know. If you aren't able to tap into your own inner guidance, return to this book and read it again. These concepts work if you dig in and give yourself the chance to change. Truly changing the core beliefs that have been holding you back takes time. Give yourself a chance to grow. But most important of all, pay attention to the process and learn to appreciate the journey.

PRIME

PART THREE

FIT BODY

It is the mind that makes the body.
—SOJOURNER TRUTH

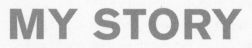

MY STORY

Earlier I wrote that once I stopped competing as an athlete, I had a difficult time maintaining my workouts. In my mind, training
was an all-or-nothing proposition. I knew
that I didn't want to build or maintain a big
physique any longer, so I stopped training
with all-out intensity in order to let my muscles shrink to more "normal" dimensions,
envisioning a time when I would replace my
all-out training with a more reasonable
approach. But I didn't seem to drift naturally
toward training at a lower, more sustainable
intensity level.

For several years I seemed to get away with this. My natural body—in addition to the residual impact of many years of training—kept me from feeling too far out of shape. That was fine until one day, around the age of 38, I noticed that my body *was* changing. I saw a snapshot of myself taken at the beach and I looked . . . different. Maybe even a touch saggy. I had already been dealing with steady decreases in my flexibility and endurance. My body seemed to be sore all the time, even though I hadn't worked out. That's when I had a good talk with myself and really faced the fact that, if I didn't do something soon, middle age was going to sneak up on me and the battle would only grow more difficult with each passing sedentary year. I went back to my workouts, but with a whole different approach—the one I take in this book, which I consider to be holistic in nature. I wasn't after the huge, ultra-defined muscles of my peak competitive years; I was pursuing the most athletic, strong, and balanced body I could build without letting the workouts take over my life. I wanted plenty of muscle to keep my metabolism stoked as a fat-burning machine, holding the creeping spread of middle age from taking permanent hold. I wanted to have great endurance, but also to keep my heart and lungs in great shape to forestall any future health issues. Most important, though, I realized that I was at a point in my life at which my actions were having a direct impact on how healthy my later middle and senior years would be. I needed to get back on track, not only to look great and keep the flab in check, but to also prevent my long-term health from spiraling downhill through my own neglect.

THE WHOLE BODY

You walk around in a machine. If it isn't well oiled and maintained, with time it will rust. There's no way around this fact. Only through understanding the complexities of these flesh-and-blood machines can we find ways to take our maturing bodies to new levels of fitness.

My approach doesn't involve trying to convince you that you must build a championship-level physique to consider yourself in shape. On the contrary, you should be seeking ways to use the tools of exercise to make your machine run more smoothly and as a side effect come away with a better looking—and a natural looking—athletic and healthy body.

Will my approach absolutely guarantee that you'll have a "six-pack" of abdominal muscles or the strength of an ox? No. I can, however, assure you that if you follow these guidelines, you'll come away fit on the inside (holding at bay the downward spiral of disease and malady—the "rust"—that can slowly creep up on a man) as well as on the outside (looking wonderful in a bathing suit without looking as if you've spent all day and night at the gym).

You'll probably need to be willing to sacrifice a few old sacred cows about working out, though. My approach is unique. I don't think you need to scream and yell your way through 400-pound bench-presses to achieve a nice body. Leave all that to the uninformed, less-mature guys who have nothing better to do with their time. It's time to evolve to something better.

I'll guide you to really focus in on how your body responds to exercise—especially once the capacity for easy gains and quick recuperation of youth has faded. Many of us grow up thinking that exercise is all about slinging as much weight around a gym as possible, or sprinting around a track trying to outrun the competition. That's certainly OK for some, but it's pretty terrible for the average 40+ body. You want your workouts to contribute to the quality of your life, not destroy it.

As with the MOTIVATED MIND, the FIT BODY is comprised of several important elements. To create a truly FIT BODY, you should strive to:

Respect Your Body

Develop Muscle

Strengthen Your Heart and Lungs

Build Flexibility

Create Proper Routines

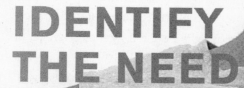

IDENTIFY
THE NEED

I prize even the failures and disillusionments, which are but steps toward success.
—MAHATMA GANDHI

Here are a few examples of challenges and hurdles that may stand between a 40+ man and a truly FIT BODY. Remember that while many of these challenges may sound "negative," we must first name something to claim it. *Identify the need* first, then seek an informed solution. See if you can identify some of your own needs below. Also, give some consideration to what your own particular fitness needs may be.

- A man slowly stops being physically active as time passes.

- He allows his body to decline, telling himself that it is inevitable.

- He believes that because of this decline and the habit of inaction, it is too late to change.

- He looks in the mirror and sees the droop where once he was solid.

- His strength has diminished in ways that sometimes surprise him.

- He avoids going anyplace where he might not be fully clothed.

- He's easily winded just climbing some stairs or walking.

- His lack of any sustained activity is causing his fat levels to creep up.

- His pulse races even when he's sitting still.

- He can't bend over and touch his toes without pain.

- His joints are constantly achy.

- He has limitations in his range of physical mobility that weren't there in his younger days.

- He holds himself back because his understanding of exercise is limited.

- He feels that with enough sit-ups he can lose his gut.

- He believes, or acts as if, his body needs no exercise to stay healthy.

- He thinks the only way to train is to throw tons of weight around in the gym.

- He has never developed the link between his mind and his muscles.

- He doesn't understand how exercises really work, and he pays no attention to proper exercise form.

- He can't sustain any focus while exercising.

- His efforts lack energy.

- His body takes twice as long to recover from strenuous activity as it did in his youth.

- He thinks that he must work out every day for many hours to get his body in shape.

- He aches whenever he does anything physical.

- He has no true understanding of how to develop an exercise routine.

- His efforts at exercise are erratic and disorganized.

- He wanders around the gym feeling lost, but pretending to be better informed than he is.

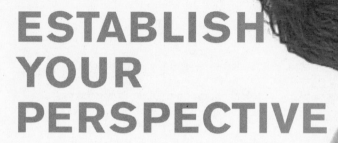

ESTABLISH
YOUR
PERSPECTIVE

It's time to play 20 Questions again, so you can have a deeper understanding of what your current beliefs are in relation to developing your own FIT BODY. As you did in MOTIVATED MIND, I strongly encourage you to write down your answers and further observations in your journal. Do this exercise when you have plenty of time to focus. Breathe yourself into a nice, relaxed place, and really give yourself the chance to honestly explore where you are with these issues.

Please remember that my approach to this is unique. You shouldn't view these questions as a test on which you can get something right or wrong. This is an exercise in self-consideration. The answers that you come up with should give you insight into where you are and how you feel. They are essentially more meditation points than anything concrete.

After you've given the following 20 questions due consideration, I encourage you to bring that more enlightened perspective to the next sections—which will then hopefully help your knowledge grow and evolve.

QUESTION 1: How do you—right now, in this moment—feel about your body?

QUESTION 2: Are you in better or worse physical condition than you were ten years ago?

QUESTION 3: Do you—at any level—avoid looking at your body in the mirror?

QUESTION 4: If you could change one aspect of your current physical condition, what would it be?

QUESTION 5: In your last answer, did you name something that is within your power to change?

QUESTION 6: How much do you really understand about exercise?

QUESTION 7: Do you have any hesitation about learning new and better techniques?

QUESTION 8: In a practical, everyday way, do you feel strong?

QUESTION 9: Do you think that you can get rid of fat by doing sit-ups?

QUESTION 10: Has your ability to recover from physical activity lessened recently?

QUESTION 11: If you had to put together an exercise routine, could you?

QUESTION 12: Do you know how your muscles work?

QUESTION 13: Do you feel as if you are overweight?

QUESTION 14: What is your training experience?

QUESTION 15: What do you hope to achieve from your workouts?

QUESTION 16: How has your body traditionally responded to exercise?

QUESTION 17: What is the current state of your overall health?

QUESTION 18: When was your last complete physical?

QUESTION 19: Do you have any long-term physical challenges that you need to take into account when developing an exercise plan?

QUESTION 20: Using your recollection of your past experience as a guide, how well does your body respond to exercise?

GATHER THE FACTS

Shallow men believe in luck. I believe in cause and effect.
—RALPH WALDO EMERSON

RESPECT YOUR BODY

Your body is composed of thousands of systems either working or not working simultaneously throughout your lifetime. The systems of your body work together in a synergistic fashion: muscle strength means little without endurance; endurance is useless without the flexibility to move freely.

If you want to get in, and stay in, the best shape possible—given your genetics, goals, and potential investment—you must also respect your individuality. While your body is certainly similar to the bodies of other men, it is also highly unique.

How do you go about respecting the individuality of your body? First of all, get to know exactly how your body functions. I'm not talking about becoming obsessed with in-depth physiology; you don't need a doctorate in anatomy to get in shape. You must, however, have a broad understanding of how things work. You should know how each individual body part works, and then how each is integrated in the entire system. How else will you know how to structure your workouts? You should understand why certain movements do certain things; why aerobics and flexibility are so essential to the total fitness picture. How else can you balance all the elements that comprise total fitness?

It's very valuable to gain an understanding of how all the systems of your body work together. With that knowledge, you'll be able to go deeper into your fitness goals. And that is the road to long-term, positive habit-building. By developing this sort of understanding, you counteract the slow or nonexistent results of guesswork.

Through beginning your fitness efforts with a respect for your own body, you take control of your goals and create the greatest possible outcome for all your efforts and investment.

Another way to respect both your body and your individuality is through an informed understanding of the ratio of invested effort to desired outcome. With any fitness program, you'll achieve results in direct proportion to your invested efforts. No matter what your goals, if you skip your workouts, you won't make gains. Train with focus and energy, and you'll get to your goal. It's a simple cause-and-effect equation. So, if your goal is to build a great body, you have to be willing to invest the needed effort into that goal. If your goal is to become as fit and healthy as possible without letting the effort take over your life, then your commitment is a less-intense effort—but you'll still need to do your work. Again—no investment, no effort, no gain.

Concerning this notion of respecting our bodies, it's necessary to address an issue that has grown more prevalent in recent years. In our culture, we're constantly being bombarded with magazine and television images that make most men feel physically inadequate. Women have faced this for decades, and it's now a growing issue with men as the advertisers learn how to play on common desires and insecurities. It's important for us to fight against this—at least in our minds. The cover model on the typical men's fitness magazine works very hard—at what is essentially a full-time job—to appear fat-free and buffed for the photo shoot. I can tell you from my own experience that the way those men look in the fitness photos is a very temporary condition lasting only a week, a day, or maybe only the length of the photo session. There are only a handful of men on the planet who walk around every day looking like that. The model gets himself into this condition by tightening his diet (sometimes quite severely) and using other, more esoteric techniques that have very little to do with everyday, real-world life. Fitness-magazine-cover shape is not a standard that men—especially 40+ men—should be measuring themselves against, unless they are genetically gifted, have been consistent, longtime athletes, or want to invest many hours each day in creating a "perfect" body.

I fight against this in my own head—this notion of what having a "perfect" body means. It is a balancing act for all of us. We should strive to take care of ourselves and be fit, but we should also be very careful about what images we allow to influence our perception of what it means to be "perfect."

Here is my take on this: The notion of superficial perfection in bodies is nonsense that leads many on a road to great frustration.

For the sake of giving this concept a definition, though, I will say that the perfection a man should strive for is a deeper understanding of himself and a greater commitment to taking care of his health. A man's body isn't just perfect because he has no body fat, amazing abs, and big arms. Your body will become "perfect" when you strive to create long-term, healthy habits. Everything else is a marketing gimmick with no deeper purpose than to feed on our insecurities and make us buy things that we don't really need.

So, please respect your own body, even as you work to put your fitness habits totally on track.

DEVELOP MUSCLES

When a man tries to manage his weight, he must concentrate on two completely interconnected areas: nutrition and exercise. If you imagine your body as a machine, food is the fuel, and your muscles are the engines that drive everything.

The 40+ man should be most concerned about the loss of muscle mass and strength that comes with aging. This is the time to set into motion the habits that will keep the muscular structure sound for a lifetime.

There is no reason why a man who is 40+ can't have the muscle tone of a much younger man. The catch is that the younger man might be able to take those muscles of his for granted, while the older man will have to work at his. But that's a lot like the difference between money that's given to you and money that you work hard to earn: If you look at it from the proper perspective, you're bound to have greater appreciation for what your work has earned, and that will motivate further hard work that will create even more positive results; in other words, the work creates satisfaction and drives outcome.

In putting his FIT BODY on track, the 40+ man must first emphasize his muscular system. Building huge muscles is unnecessary; building desired strength and tone, on the other hand, will drive the metabolism and—when it's blended with good nutrition—help keep body fat, as well as premature aging and associated health problems, at bay. This is a fact that many men don't understand. While the old mythology about unused muscles turning to flab is completely false—since muscle and fat are completely different chemical compounds, and one cannot become the other—muscular development will cause the body to more efficiently burn calories and therefore burn off fat. The complex reason for this can be explained in a simple way: Muscle burns more energy than does fat. The fatter you are, the more you store fat. The more muscular you are, the more fat you burn. The direct road to a better metabolism—and therefore less overall, long-term body fat—is through increased muscle mass.

You don't need to become an obsessed gym-rat to benefit from this concept. Simply creating a system in which your muscles are stimulated and an environment for them to grow stronger is enough. But it is wise to begin by truly understanding how your muscles work.

Since we're working with a machine (the body) comprised of numerous components (including the individual parts of the "engine," your muscles), we should begin by looking at the body one component at a time. For the sake of simplicity, let's categorize the individual muscle groups like this:

- Chest

- Back

- Shoulders

- Biceps

- Triceps

- Forearms

- Front Thighs

- Hamstrings

- Calves

- Abdominals

As I said earlier, most men grow up believing that all there is to muscle-building is going off to a gym and pumping as much weight as they can. This is the worst possible way for anyone, much less a 40+ man, to train. While developing muscles isn't as complicated as, say, building a rocket ship, it does benefit a man to know what he's doing, so that he can make his workouts more efficient and avoid injuries—both vitally important issues for the 40+ man.

When approaching exercise of any type, it's good to understand that the components of your body (those individual muscle-groups listed earlier) function synergistically. In other words, the components are combined and become cooperative, and because of that, their combined output is greater than that of the sum of the parts. How does that apply to developing muscles? In the area of muscular strength, we can look at specific synergistic systems. The chest muscles, for example, require support muscles to work properly. If the chest is the primary (or targeted) muscle for an exercise, it is synergistically supported by the triceps, deltoids, and forearms, which not only play supportive roles, but also receive secondary benefit from the chest exercise. It is similar for every other body part as well. The body may be composed of individual muscles, but each of those is an important player in a larger system.

Just as the muscles are comprised of complementary, synergistic systems, so is the very means of building those muscles. In working the muscles, there are five important concepts that must be understood and put into action. And, as with the body parts themselves, each of these concepts works synergistically with the others to develop those muscles. The concepts are:

1. Resistance

2. Stimulation

3. Performance

4. Intensity

5. Recuperation

Resistance

Any time you push or pull against an object or force, you are using resistance. An object *resists* your efforts to move it, and you use your muscular strength to do so. At the risk of oversimplifying: Your muscles grow stronger by pushing or pulling against some sort of resistance. Muscles adapt to the resistance that is provided, and therefore—assuming that other key criteria are met—they grow in size and in strength. Resistance can come in a variety of forms, ranging from a dead weight to your own body. *Prime* exercises and routines will be comprised of exercises using both of these forms of resistance, namely, weight-training exercises and isometric exercises. Each of these forms of resistance training has its own significant benefits for the 40+ man.

Weight training, with barbells, dumbbells, and weight machines, will make up a large part of many of the *Prime* routines. For building greater muscular size and strength, nothing beats working against the resistance of a progressive amount of dead weight. The term *progressive* means that the weights can be lowered or raised according to the desired intensity and repetition range; one can adapt the load of the resistance in accordance with one's needs.

There is some confusion (especially among those who have little weight-training experience) regarding which is superior: free weights or weight machines. Many experts have created something of a false debate over this issue by siding with one type of equipment or the other. This is silly. A balanced approach to working out will utilize both free weights and machines. There are only minor differences between the two. All that you're trying to do with any resistance exercise is give your muscles a load to work against. It doesn't matter whether that load comes from a machine or a free weight, or even from the weight of your own body (as with a push-up).

Besides, it's nearly impossible to avoid using a mix of machinery for any good weight-training program. Machines keep the body supported during an exercise; they make the exercise very stable and therefore may provide a potential avenue to greater focus and better exercise form. On the other hand, free weights bring into play various smaller supporting muscles in order to balance the weight during the performance of an exercise. When you're doing a Barbell Bench Press, the bar must be balanced as the exercise is performed, and this balancing causes the synergistic system of supportive muscles to branch out beyond the chest, shoulders, and triceps; the effort to balance causes a flexing of smaller surrounding muscles, which can be good, but one also runs the risk of injury if technique is sloppy. That said, if you use the exercise-perfection advice that's coming up, even your free-weight exercises should be very stable and safe. So, if for example you compare a Barbell Bench Press against a Machine Chest Press, the movements are nearly identical, and the manner in which the chest muscles are stimulated is also very similar, with slight variation. One is not superior to the other. All that any type of resistance exercise attempts to do is duplicate the body's natural movements against as much of a resistance load as is needed for stimulation. For example, the Barbell Bench Press represents and duplicates one of the main functions of how the chest muscles move and work in everyday life—what their purpose is: pushing something away from the body. There are many ways to accomplish that task for each and every body part.

The second type of resistance that you'll be using in many of the *Prime* routines is my own version of *isometrics*. This is a process of using the resistance provided by your own body as the load to work against.

I especially love isometrics because they can be done anywhere with no more equipment needed than one's own body (and perhaps a simple towel for some of the exercises). While weights can improve size and strength like nothing else, isometrics are great for developing muscle tone. Essentially, the core of an isometric exercise is flexing the muscle and holding that tension for a certain amount of time. Isometrics are fantastic for a man who wants to get in shape but doesn't want to develop an overly muscular body. The isometric exercises outlined in this book are also great compliments to weight and flexibility exercises. My unique version of isometrics may be performed in either a static fashion (as in simply holding a muscle flexed for a certain amount of time) or with movement involved (as will be illustrated in the How the Muscles Work section).

Stimulation

While each muscle group is unique in its practical functions, all the muscles are stimulated in the same basic way. With weight training, the goal is much more than simply to move a weight from Point A to Point B. (The same principle applies to isometrics.) The goal is stimulating, and thus increasing strength in, a body part by alternately shortening and lengthening the muscle being primarily focused upon against the resistance of the applied load, be that a weight, the body, or static tension.

Just as there is a perfect golf swing—where everything is sweet and the ball goes exactly where it should—so too does each muscle have a perfect pathway of movement that it must follow for the exercise to be properly executed. Anyone who does any form of resistance training should be intimately familiar and respectful of proper muscle pathways; however, for the 40+ man, this familiarity is absolutely essential. As the body ages, its tendency to get injured by sloppy exercise form increases dramatically. Whereas a younger man might (but really shouldn't) get away with terrible exercise form mainly due to the sheer resilience of his young body, the average 40+ man can't; the older man may well (and often does) become injured by using poor exercise technique. A young body will generally rebound from simple injuries, whereas an older body will take much longer to heal.

In order for each muscle to be stimulated, it must be contracted—in other words, flexed, or clenched with strong tension. Then it must travel along its perfect pathway to its opposite position. The opposite of the contracted position is the stretch—in which the muscle is fully extended. You can see this more clearly if you look at the biceps muscles of your arm. When your elbow is extended and the arm is straight, the biceps muscles are stretched. When the elbow is bent so that the hand comes toward the shoulder, the biceps muscles are in a shortened, or flexed, position. It is similar with every muscle throughout your body. Each has a lengthened (or stretched) position and a shortened (or flexed) position. Take another example: the push-up, which primarily stimulates the chest muscles. While your body acts as the force of resistance, when your arms are bent and your chest is against the floor, the muscles of your chest are fully stretched. In opposition to the stretch, the chest is flexed (or contracted) when you are at the top of the movement—arms fully extended, upper body pushed away from the floor.

In any resistance exercise, one journey along the muscle's pathway, from stretch to contraction and back again, is a *repetition*. A *set* is made up of a certain number of repetitions (or *reps* for short). If you do ten reps and stop, that's a set.

Simply put, stretching and contracting a muscle over and over again (in repetitions and sets) against resistance is what stimulates it to respond—to grow stronger and larger.

Just as each individual muscle has a different mechanical function, each also has the need for a variety of repetition schemes for stimulation. I've often been asked if I believe in using heavy weights during a workout. My answer is generally yes—with a fairly large asterisk attached. First, we must decide what is meant by "a heavy weight." After all, a weight that seems like nothing to one man will be impossible to move for another.

I've always defined a heavy weight as being one that, while using absolutely perfect exercise form and working toward the desired number of reps, takes the muscles to positive failure. I'll discuss this concept of positive failure more in the upcoming sections on Performance and Intensity, but for the moment, let me say that positive failure occurs when, at the end of a set of an exercise, one more repetition is not possible without either a break in perfect form (such as the use of momentum—in other words, "cheating") or the addition of outside assistance to help move the weight (what's known as getting a *forced rep*). Positive failure occurs after the last repetition that you can do all by yourself using perfect exercise form.

When stimulating the muscles to grow you must work them in a variety of repetition ranges. There is something of a mythology attached to weight training that says that only low numbers of repetitions are needed to cause muscles to grow. This is only true in part. The whole truth is that the muscle fibers are stimulated by performing exercises in the low-, medium-, and high-repetition ranges; each of these has its benefits.

Low repetitions (6 to 10 per set) help strengthen the muscle fibers as well as the tendons and ligaments. Low repetitions build a foundation of core strength. I would also note here that, in terms of general fitness, doing sets with fewer than 6 repetitions is counterproductive. For many men, it's very difficult to break out of the old-fashioned mindset of seeing how much they can bench-press, for example, for a single repetition. But from a fitness-and-development standpoint (especially for any man over 40), this is an exercise in ego that can lead only to an extreme vulnerability to injury. Single-repetition sets lead nowhere positive in the context of a *Prime* program and must be avoided.

Medium repetitions (10 to 15 per set) are most responsible for building muscle tone and mass in the majority of each muscle's fibers.

High repetitions (15 or more per set) build endurance fibers of the muscle known as mitochondria; these particular fibers compose up to 25 percent of muscle mass in some body parts.

For truly balanced development, I design programs with a variety of repetition schemes. Contrary to what many trainers and other experts might say, your body needs a great deal of variety to achieve maximum fitness. In my routines, the exceptions to this rule lie in many of the beginner programs and in those oriented more toward tone than toward muscle size and strength. For these programs, I generally use higher repetition ranges. This is to develop a greater mind-muscle link.

Performance

The mind-muscle link is a neurological pathway that is developed with experience in progressively contracting muscles during resistance exercise. Essentially, it is learning to feel the muscles work through a combination of strict form, mental concentration, and well-executed repetitions—all of which combine, in another of those synergistic systems, to create a heightened outcome. To develop a muscle, it is essential to feel it work. This is a fact either not known, or ignored, by huge numbers of men who work out. It really is the manifestation of the false notion—which bears repeating in order to reinforce how counterproductive it is—that all there is to weight training is slinging a bunch of weights around, perhaps even carrying on a conversation while doing so. And as I have already said a few times, since it is so central to my training philosophies, this is not the path to efficiently achieving fitness goals. If not, what is? Three things that have to do with performance:

- Feeling the muscles work

- Exercise perfection

- Proper repetition performance

Each of these three concepts is completely interrelated with the others. Blending them together is the fastest road to exercise success that I know. In fact, these may well be some of the most important concepts of detail in the entire FIT BODY part of the book.

Exercise is a tactile experience, and this is especially true of resistance exercise. To make it work, you've got to feel it work. This essentially means that when you're performing any exercise, whether the resistance is weight or isometric tension, as your repetitions travel along their perfect pathway (like the perfect and sweet golf swing), your attention should be so tuned in to the muscle that you feel it burn as it stretches and burn even more as you flex it into a contraction. Notice that I've once again returned to this concept of *attention*? Do you see how important a role this concept of paying attention plays in creating fitness success? When you do your exercises, don't simply go through the motions. Don't make the mistake of reading that some aspect of a routine calls for 15 repetitions and then rush through them as if they're a nasty chore instead of an investment in efficiently developing a better body—as well as an exercise in mental focus. Instead, feel the muscle work through each rep and every set—through the entire workout.

If you're like me, you want the time that you spend exercising to have maximum benefit. If you want the muscle to respond, you've got to feel it work. By doing this, you develop that mind-muscle link that I mentioned earlier, which runs from the brain down the nerves and into the muscles, forging a direct response pathway.

The best way to go about this also requires attention to detail. I'm an absolute believer in learning what I call exercise perfection. This is essentially similar to that sweet zone found in any physical activity (that perfect golf swing, or the form used to bowl a perfect strike). Just as each muscle has a perfect performance pathway from stretch to contraction and back again, there's a perfect manner in which each exercise should be performed. That means not throwing the weights around. It means slowing everything down. Imagine the difference between rushing through something important and taking your time with it. When you do an exercise, you want essentially to center your energy, slow yourself down, direct your full attention to the task at hand, and feel the exercise work by performing every repetition with perfect form.

The best way I know of to combine exercise feel with exercise perfection is to stop focusing on how much weight is on the bar. Weight is, to a large extent, kind of irrelevant. I know that in some weight-training circles this is considered blasphemous; however, I've used these very concepts throughout my career and not only achieved great success with them but also remained injury-free. Here's an important piece of advice: Never worry whether or not you appear to be the strongest man in the gym. You are training for yourself only. Work to perfect your focus and technique, and you will be the man who makes the dramatic change. So, if weight isn't important, what is? The way that you do each repetition, that's what.

Slow the repetitions down. Way down. That's how your muscles will respond. Your maturing muscles will not respond well to fast, sloppy repetitions. That is an open invitation to injury, not to mention a lack of results. Instead, I'd like you to imagine resistance exercises as more of an active meditative process. By that, I mean that I want you to exert absolute and slow control over the way you do your exercises. That means taking your time. The travel time from stretch to contraction should be a minimum of three to four seconds. That means that if you're doing a Barbell Curl for your biceps, from the stretch (where your arms are fully extended) to the contraction (where the bar is curled and the biceps are flexed against the resistance) you should be so much in control of the weight that you take at least three to four seconds to get there. Then you should lower the weight in the same manner. Don't just drop it back to the stretch. Resist. Better yet, when the muscle is in the flexed position, take at least a two-count and really flex that muscle hard—really feel as if you're squeezing the muscle with tension. You should do this on every exercise, every set. It will feel as if you are moving in slow motion, but it will revolutionize your workouts. This is important. You will see very few men training this way; most perform their reps and sets in a fast, sloppy, jerky manner. Ignore them. They aren't doing it right.

Training this way takes attention and focus. It will not be easy. It is, however, a tremendously effective manner of training. I'll use slow and squeezing repetitions in all the routines described later in the book.

Intensity

As I mentioned before, in the discussion of intensity in exercise, ground zero is this concept of positive failure, in which the last repetition you do in a set is the last one that you can possibly do without getting assistance or breaking good form. You must use a certain level of intense focus and physical effort to make sure that positive failure is truly all you can give, within the parameters given above.

Intensity, in the context of exercise, means the amount of energy that you put into the activity. When building a program for fitness, you'll need to exercise with some degree of intensity; otherwise, no stimulation will occur. If you do a Bench-Press set and perform five disinterested reps when, with a bit of focus and energy, you could have done 20, the lack of intensity will mean that your muscle stimulation will be minimal. Exercise intensity should be adjusted according to need. If you are an absolute beginner or are just returning to exercise after a long time away, break yourself in with less-intense workouts. Nothing discourages a beginner more than starting out all gung-ho and then getting extremely sore and tired from the first few workouts. In fact, this is one of the reasons that so many men quit soon after starting. So, adjust your workout intensity accordingly. Not too much, not too little. How will you know the difference? Listen to your body (as I'll discuss further in the Recuperation section); it has an amazing way of giving you direct feedback.

If halfhearted effort and a lack of focus lead to too little intensity, what constitutes too much? Intensity is too great when it pushes the body past its normal capacity to recover from the exercise in a reasonable amount of time. This generally happens for one of the following reasons:

1. The overall energy output is too great.

2. The duration of the workout is too long.

3. The volume of exercise is too high.

4. Too much emphasis is placed on going beyond positive failure.

In the Create Routines section, I'll delve deeper into the duration-and-volume issue. In general, however, while exercise performance and repetitions should be slow, workout duration and volume (the number of exercises and sets) should be relatively brief. No workout should ever take longer than an hour. My own weight workouts rarely last longer than 45 minutes, because they are focused and intense. I don't spend social time during my training. I take the absolutely briefest rest periods between sets. I get the work done and then let it go. So should you. Long workouts are only for those who don't have anything better to do than be in the gym, and for those who don't want to make maximum gains.

There are several techniques that are used to push an exercise beyond positive failure.

Some of them are of value—if you know how and when to use them. Some of them should be avoided.

1. Forced repetitions: This is perhaps the most abused intensity technique in all of weight training. The idea is that another person helps you lift the weight when it gets too heavy for you to do any more reps with good form. Ideally, a training partner helps by lifting a fraction of the weight on the last rep or two of an intense set, helping the lifter to squeeze out just a bit more stimulation than he would be able to do on his own. However, this is a very misunderstood technique. It is generally abused when a man uses more weight than he can realistically handle during a set and has his partner help him on several reps—maybe even every rep of the whole set. Sometimes, training partners will try to get someone to do forced reps just to try to push the intensity. While this is usually well-intended, it is a mistake to do very many forced repetitions. They push the body past its own ability to recover from the training. As I'll discuss in a moment, this issue of recovery is an important one to the 40+ man. Forced repetitions should be used only by the most advanced trainers and only very sparingly.

2. Drop sets: These work in a way quite similar to forced reps. A set is done to positive failure, and then the weight is put down. Immediately and without rest, a slightly lighter weight is picked up and the same exercise is done, again to positive failure. A second and third drop can also be added. Perfect exercise form must be maintained during a drop set since, as the muscle grows fatigued, it is easy to get sloppy and open the body up to injury. This is a very advanced technique that should only be used sparingly, since it pushes the body far past its normal recuperation abilities. If abused, it will have an effect opposite to the intended one. It will keep the body part from improving, because the muscles won't recover.

3. Multiple sets (*super-sets, bi-sets, tri-sets, giant sets*): This is a combination of two or more exercises done with very little rest, one after the other. A super-set is a combination of two exercises, each of which is for a different body part. A super-set might have a chest exercise combined with a back exercise. A bi-set is a combination of two exercises done one right after the other for the same body part. For example, two leg exercises done consecutively with little or no rest between them is a bi-set. Their combination would be treated as one set, with any rest coming at the end of the bi-set. A tri-set is similar in structure to a bi-set, but it consists of three exercises for the same body part. A giant-set is four or more exercises for the same body part with little or no rest between them.

These techniques—especially in a weight-training routine—are generally used in more advanced workouts, although there will be some exceptions. They have the advantage of shortening the length of a workout because of decreased rest time, but they also push the body very hard and seriously tax the recuperative abilities.

4. Cheating: This is a break in perfect exercise form. It is usually done for two reasons, one bad and the other good only in a way similar to the way that forced reps can be good. The bad reason is rooted in poor exercise form. I've already emphasized my philosophy about not using sloppy form. For the 40+ man, poorly utilized cheating will likely lead to injuries that may sidetrack the entire program. Use exercise perfection instead. The "good" form of cheating would more accurately be called controlled cheating. It is a very advanced technique in which the lifter uses a bit (and I emphasize *a bit*) of body momentum to achieve a last rep or two in an intense set in order to push past positive failure. For example, a man wants to get another rep in a set of Barbell Curls, but can't do it with perfect form, so he swings his body a bit to nudge the bar up over the edge of failure. Controlled cheating should only be used by those who know what they're doing, and then only sparingly and under control.

Recuperation

Without exaggeration, I can say that one of the top issues facing the 40+ man is his ability to recuperate from intense exercise. It is a simple fact of life that as the body ages, its ability to recover from vigorous activity declines. This becomes somewhat less true the more active a man is on a consistent basis, but only to a point. I don't recover as quickly from a workout now as I did when I was 25. That doesn't mean, however, that I can't adapt and compensate and keep my athletic abilities in top shape. Just as with so many other issues, I have simply had to give the issue more attention and thoughtful effort as I've aged.

Recovery is perhaps the most overlooked issue in everyday exercise philosophy. We learn how to train—even if some of the techniques aren't exactly perfect—yet we act as if that's all there is to the equation: Lift some weight, forget about it, and muscles will grow. If only it were that simple.

Progress from a workout is driven by two essential factors:

■ Stimulation (which I've already covered above)

■ Recuperation

If you don't allow your body adequate rest after stimulating it with intense exercise, it will not recover and progress will be stalled. You'll also end up quite sore and possibly injured; these are accumulated by-products in a system that has not recuperated. Exercise stimulation is a type of stress, and just as you need rest to recover from other stressors, so too does your exercised body need rest to renew itself.

The balancing act in creating a fit life is to keep the elements of stimulation and recuperation working together rather than against each other. The stronger the stimulation of the body's systems is, the greater the quality and amount of recovery necessary. Stimulate too much and rest too little, and you'll burn out. Stimulate too little and rest too much, and you'll never get in shape.

Just as there are a number of ways to make sure that your body is well stimulated, there are also many techniques that the 40+ man can draw on to help him recover well from his efforts. The good news is that there are positive side effects of many of these techniques that extend beyond the workouts. And that is one of the best aspects of building a fitness and wellness program. Exercise is good for you, yes, but it also impacts the rest of your life in many positive ways, and so do well-directed recuperation techniques.

The best way to recover adequately from your workouts is to tune in to the rhythms of your own body. Again I return to this concept of *attention*, which in this situation means learning to observe the signals that your body sends you. If you're overly sore and tired after a workout, you need more rest. If you don't feel tired at all the day after training, you're either on-target or not training with enough intensity. The difference is going to be judged according to your own observations. Remember that with exercise you're trying to draw the fine line between too much and too little. Key in to your body's signals, learn what they mean, and pay attention to them.

Of course, it seems almost unnecessary to mention that the key way to recuperate is to sleep. Yet we live in a culture in which many men burn the candle at both ends and certainly don't allow their bodies enough quality sleep.

Beyond the age of 40—and especially if you become physically active—your body needs seven to eight hours of quality sleep every night. The days of getting away with little or no sleep are over. It's almost as if there's a return to the needs of childhood in this regard. To look and feel young, you cannot skip sleeping well every night. You can try taking a brief nap during the day if you're unable to get a full night of quality sleep. Try to relax and close your eyes for 10 to 20 minutes after lunch.

In fact, one of the best recuperation techniques of all is to meditate and use the positive visualization techniques discussed in MOTIVATED MIND. Return to those sections and redouble your relaxation exercises if you find yourself unable to sleep well. Guided meditation can also work to calm the mind for those unable to fall asleep easily at night.

You should also try to go to bed at a regular time each night, avoid caffeine after 4 P.M. and try to keep your sleeping environment cool (since our bodies sleep more easily under these conditions). Above all else, don't depend on alcohol or drugs to get to sleep; instead, work to organically relax your mind. Alcohol-induced sleep is not restful sleep. And you should be teaching your body natural ways to relax in order to achieve not just better-quality rest, but also a greater sense of overall health.

If your muscles aren't recovering adequately from your workouts, I recommend that you try four additional techniques:

1. Immediately after the workout, use an ice pack on any particularly sore muscles.

2. Take a long, hot bath, and meditate. Do your positive visualizations as you soak away the soreness.

3. Stretch your muscles in a relaxed way (which I'll cover in greater depth in a moment).

4. Massage the muscles that you've been working. Self-massage helps speed the recovery process and also helps you understand more about your own body—where it gets tight and stiff, where it gets particularly sore. Just use your own fingertips to dig into those sore, tight spots. This is especially helpful after a hot bath and stretching.

Finally, if you find that you aren't recovering adequately, use one of the various forms of massage that are available. If massaging our own muscles is helpful on a regular basis, then getting a professional massage is like taking an intense recovery pill.

THE POWER OF MASSAGE

Massage therapy has been around for as long as three thousand years. Having a professional massage doesn't just feel great; it helps the body recover from intense exercise, and there are many more health-related reasons for a 40+ man to indulge in periodic or regular massage therapy, which:

- Helps reduce stress in both mind and body

- Releases muscle tension

- Stimulates better circulation

- Induces mental relaxation

- Removes toxins to promote overall healing

- Allows for greater flexibility and ease of movement

- Improves interrelationships between bodily systems

In addition, massage therapy acts in a holistic and healing manner to help integrate aspects of the body and mind and is commonly used to address a variety of conditions, such as:

- Back pain

- Tension headaches

- Sleep disorders

- Anxiety

- Depression

- Hypertension

- Job-related stress

- Rheumatoid arthritis

A few words of caution: Given the number of people who hang out a shingle and call themselves massage therapists (it's estimated that there are fifty thousand massage therapist's practicing in the U.S. alone), find someone who is licensed and experienced in the style of massage that you seek. Currently, 29 states and the District of Columbia regulate the profession and ensure that a licensed massage therapist meets the 500-hour standard set by the Commission on Massage Therapy.

Select the type of massage that best suits your needs.

TYPE	PROCEDURE	BENEFIT	LENGTH	COST
SWEDISH	Gliding, kneading strokes and tapping or shaking are used to relax muscles and loosen joints.	relaxation, boost circulation, reduce swelling from injury, and boost immune system	usually 30–90 minutes	typically $30–$100/hour
SPORTS MASSAGE	A variation of Swedish massage but with more intensity as direct pressure is used to reduce muscle spasms.	speed recovery of sore muscles, increase range of motion, protect from workout-related injuries if used proactively	usually 30–60 minutes	same as above
TRIGGER POINT (MYOTHERAPY)	Finger pressure is used to release chronically tight muscles caused by overtraining, trauma, or poor posture.	ease lower back pain, relieve tension headaches and other body discomfort caused by tense muscles	usually 60 minutes	same as above
SHIATSU (ACUPRESSURE)	The therapist uses hands, elbows, knees, and feet to apply pressure to points on the body believed to be connected to the body's internal organs.	unblock a life force the Chinese refer to as *Qi* (pronounced Chee) or what some Westerners believe to be the release of endorphins, the body's natural painkillers	usually 30–90 minutes	same as above
MYOFASCIAL RELEASE	The therapist uses fingers, palms, and elbows to stretch your fascia (soft connective tissue located between muscle and bone) with long, firm strokes lasting between 90 seconds and several minutes.	reduce pain and stiffness caused when fascia tightens up and pulls muscles out of place; used to treat chronic pain	usually 30–90 minutes	same as above
ROLFING	Deep, often painful pressure is applied with fingers, forearms, and elbows to realign fascia.	relieve chronic pain and improve flexibility caused by poor alignment of fascia due to accidents, posture, and emotional stress	usually done in a series of 10 sessions, each session lasting 60–90 minutes	usually $75–$125/ session

HOW THE MUSCLES WORK

The final aspect that ties all of these concepts together is a full knowledge of how each muscle actually works. Most of your muscles have more than one function. Each muscle can be exercised from a variety of angles pertaining to each of its functions. Listed below are: each body part with its function, an example exercise, and that exercise's stretch and contraction points. I've also given additional examples of exercises that work the various angles of the muscle for each function. While this isn't a list of every exercise imaginable for each body part, many of those listed will be exercises used in various *Prime* routines.

CHEST

FUNCTION #1: PRESSING MOVEMENTS

Pushing the body away from something or pushing something away from the body.

EXAMPLE EXERCISE

Flat Dumbbell Bench Press (for the mid-chest)

STRETCH

The dumbbells are lowered until they are near the armpits, and the elbows are pulled back so that they are directly under the hands.

CONTRACTION

The arms are fully extended, with the load of the weight supported by the flexed chest muscles.

Stretch Position
for Flat Dumbbell
Bench Press

Contraction Position
for Flat Dumbbell
Bench Press

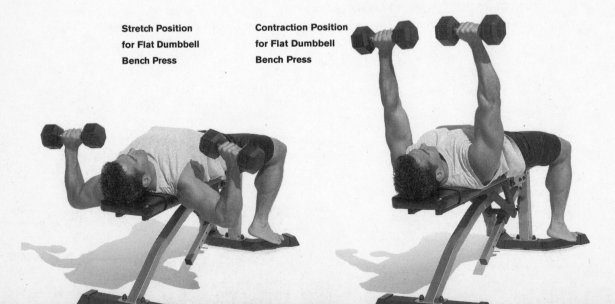

Additional Chest Pressing Exercises

OTHER DUMBBELL PRESSES

If done on an incline bench (set no steeper than 45 degrees), these stimulate the upper chest (an often-neglected area). I generally structure chest workouts more around inclined movements than lying flat ones because the upper chest is hard to stimulate. I tend to avoid decline movements (lying on a slanted bench with the feet higher than the head), as they develop a heavy lower chest that can appear saggy even if it is solid.

BARBELL BENCH PRESS

These can be done either on a flat bench (for the lower and mid-chest) or on an incline bench (for the upper chest).

MACHINE PRESS

Basically similar in function to barbell and dumbbell presses. They come in variations that can duplicate a flat or inclined angle.

DIP

If done with the elbows slightly flared out and the chin tucked into the chest, the upper body rolled slightly forward, these stimulate the lower and mid-chest.

PUSH-UP

This duplicates a flat press if the feet are on the ground and the elbows are flared out away from the body. It is similar to an incline press if the feet are elevated (on a bench, for instance) and the back is kept flat and not allowed to sway downward.

FUNCTION #2: FLY MOVEMENT

Beginning with arms extended to the sides, using the chest to bring the arms across in front of the body

EXAMPLE EXERCISE

Incline Dumbbell Fly (for the upper chest)

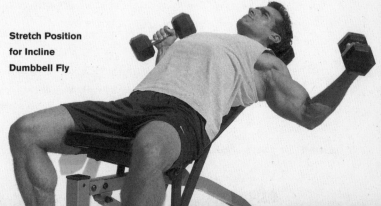

Stretch Position for Incline Dumbbell Fly

STRETCH

With the arms locked in a position with the elbows slightly bent, the weights are lowered out and away from the body to chest level.

CONTRACTION

The Weights are touching above the chest, the arms still slightly bent and the chest muscles supporting the weight load by flexing.

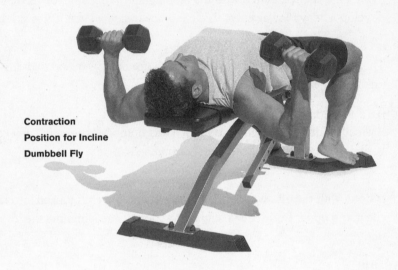

**Contraction
Position for Incline
Dumbbell Fly**

Additional Fly Movements

OTHER DUMBBELL-FLY MOVEMENTS

Flys can be done on an incline bench to work the upper chest.

MACHINES

The fly is duplicated on apparatus such as the Pec-Deck and other chest "squeezing" machines.

CABLE FLYS

Done while standing (Cable Crossovers) or while lying on a flat or incline bench, these are simply variations on the fly movement.

BACK

FUNCTION #1: PULL-UP OR PULL-DOWN MOVEMENTS

With the arms extended overhead, pulling a weight toward the body, or the body toward a suspended, stationary horizontal bar, by pulling downward, bending the arms at the elbows, and rotating the shoulder joints.

EXAMPLE EXERCISE

Wide-Grip Front Pull-Up

STRETCH

The arms are fully extended, the shoulders pulled upward from their natural position.

CONTRACTION

The entire body is pulled up, until the chest is nearly touching the stationary overhead bar, by bending the elbows and pulling back until they are in line just beneath and slightly behind the hands. The back muscles are flexed.

Additional Pull-Up/Pull-Down Movements

CHINS

Similar to Pull-Ups but done with an underhand grip. It's important to note that all pull-ups and pull-downs can be performed with a variety of grip widths. It's generally accepted that the wider the grip, the more the sides of the back are affected; the closer the grip, the more the central back is stimulated.

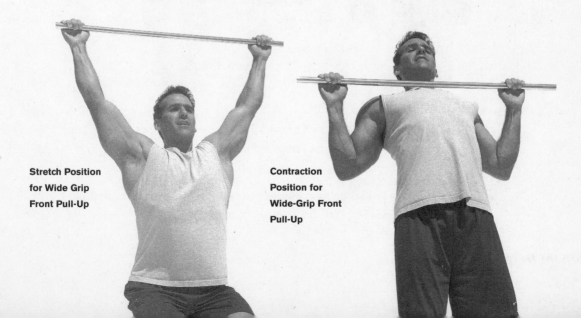

Stretch Position for Wide Grip Front Pull-Up

Contraction Position for Wide-Grip Front Pull-Up

PULL-DOWNS

From wide grip to close grip, the variety is extensive. These can also be done by pulling the bar to the chest (which should be lifted at the ribcage as if slightly arching the back) or behind the neck (this works the muscles higher on the back).

MACHINES

These simply duplicate the performance pathway of the pull-up or pulley-style pull-down.

FUNCTION #2: ROWING MOVEMENTS

Pulling weight toward the body from a position directly in front of the upper torso.

EXAMPLE EXERCISE

Two-Dumbbell Row

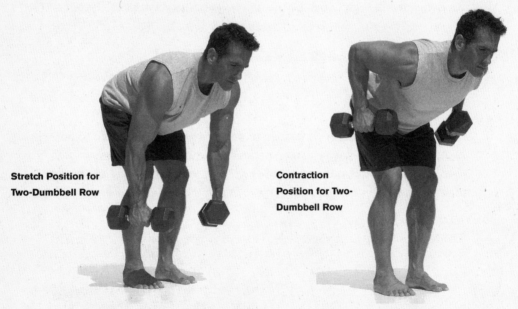

Stretch Position for Two-Dumbbell Row

Contraction Position for Two-Dumbbell Row

STRETCH

The arms are stretched down toward the ground, the upper body is bent forward at the waist, and the knees are slightly bent.

CONTRACTION

The hands are pulled up to the sides near the hips; the elbows are pulled back as far as possible; the back muscles are flexed.

Additional Rowing Movements

DUMBBELL

These can also be done one side at a time. Rest one bent leg on a flat bench, gripping the bench with one hand and a dumbbell in the other, and follow the above stretch-and-contraction sequence.

PULLEY MACHINE

The Low Pulley Row is a standard whole-back builder. Be sure to keep the knees slightly bent, and don't lean back to move the weight; use the back muscles to exert the force.

BARBELL ROWS

Caution must be used in this exercise, as it puts tremendous pressure on the lower back.

MACHINES

Again, these simply try to duplicate the free-weight pathways, but they can be great for perfecting form and isolating the target muscles.

FUNCTION #3: LOWER BACK MOVEMENTS

Bending and straightening at the waist, working the lower erector muscles.

EXAMPLE EXERCISE

Good Morning

STRETCH

The body is bent at the waist, the upper body stretched forward as far as possible.

CONTRACTION

The body is upright yet slightly bent forward at the waist. The lower back muscles are flexed.

Additional Lower Back Movement

HYPEREXTENSIONS

Performed on a special bench, the bending and straightening at the waist is similar to Good Mornings and safer for someone with lower-back problems. Both of these exercises are also terrific for the glutes and hamstrings.

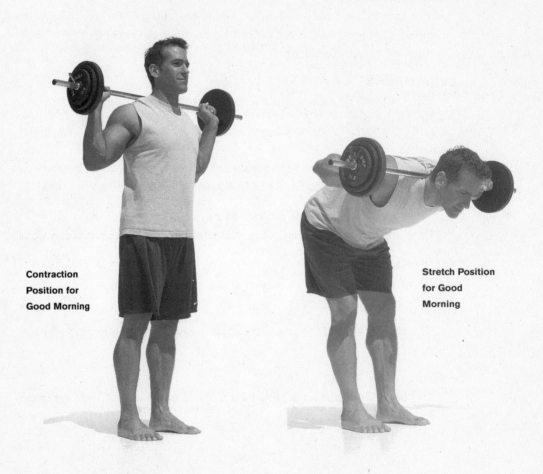

Contraction Position for Good Morning

Stretch Position for Good Morning

SHOULDERS

FUNCTION #1: PRESSING MOVEMENTS

Pushing weight away from the body overhead as opposed to in front (as in a chest press)

EXAMPLE EXERCISE

Dumbbell Press

STRETCH

The dumbbells are lowered until they are next to the shoulders; the elbows are pulled back.

CONTRACTION

The arms are extended so that the weights are up overhead; the weight is held up by the flexed shoulder muscles, not by locked-out arms; the shoulders are flexed.

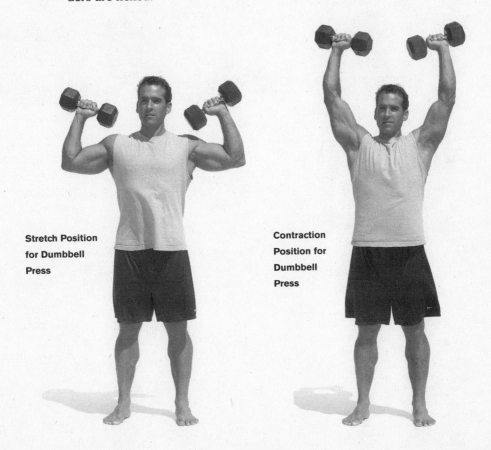

Stretch Position for Dumbbell Press

Contraction Position for Dumbbell Press

PRIME

Additional Shoulder Pressing Movements

BARBELL PRESSES

Both dumbbell and barbell presses can be done while standing (which can be hard on some men's backs) or while seated (best when the back is supported by a bench with an upright back, like the back of a chair). The barbell version of this movement can also be performed by bringing the bar either in front of the head or behind the neck. I usually prefer Behind-the-Neck Presses because they give a better shoulder stretch.

MACHINES

These duplicate the function of free weights in a way that is stable and supported.

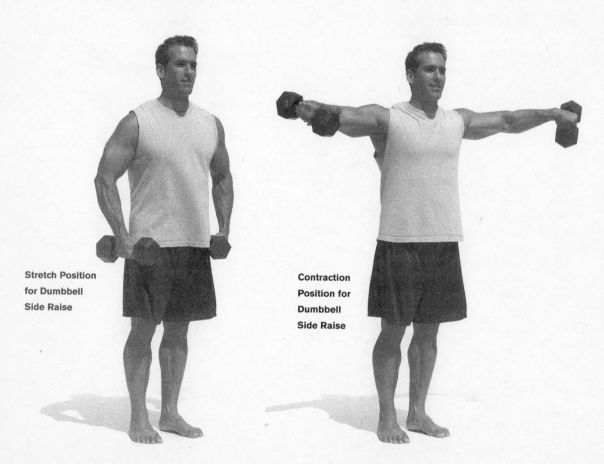

Stretch Position for Dumbbell Side Raise

Contraction Position for Dumbbell Side Raise

FUNCTION #2: LATERAL MOVEMENTS

With the arms extended to the front or sides, moving the arms up and down.

EXAMPLE EXERCISE

Dumbbell Side Raise

STRETCH

The weights and arms are along the sides of the body, the weights resting against the sides of the thighs.

CONTRACTION

The weights are out away from the body at arm's length and at shoulder height. The shoulder muscles are flexed.

Additional Lateral Movements

OTHER DUMBBELL SIDE RAISES

This exercise can be done from a variety of angles. Standing upright stimulates the sides of the deltoid muscles. Bending at the waist, whether seated or standing, and doing a lateral movement (Bent-Over Lateral Raises) affects the rear portion of the deltoids. Raising the dumbbells to the front of the body stimulates the front deltoid. (Most men don't need this movement, as the front deltoid is also heavily stimulated during Chest Press exercises and can easily be overworked and injured.)

PULLEYS AND OTHER MACHINES

Again, these duplicate the free-weight movements in a more controlled range of motion. The variety of potential angles that can be stimulated is quite large.

BICEPS

FUNCTION #1

Bringing the hand (palm facing up) and forearm toward the body by bending the elbow

EXAMPLE EXERCISE

Dumbbell Curl

STRETCH

The dumbbells are held with the palms facing forward; the arms are fully extended and the weights rest next to the thighs.

CONTRACTION

The dumbbells are raised by bending the elbows. The biceps shorten and flex.

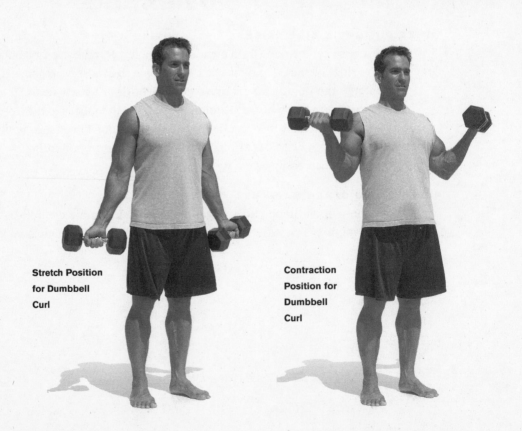

**Stretch Position
for Dumbbell
Curl**

**Contraction
Position for
Dumbbell
Curl**

Additional Biceps Curling Exercises

OTHER DUMBBELL CURLS

These can be done standing or seated, curling both arms simultaneously or curling with one arm and then the other in alternation.

BARBELL CURLS

While standing, be sure not to swing the body to help raise the barbell. Be sure also to fully extend the arms into a straight-down position during the stretch phase of this (and any other) biceps movement. Many men tend to do only partial reps, stopping before the biceps are fully stretched.

PULLEYS AND MACHINES

These duplicate the curling action in a more controlled range of motion but still should be performed with attention to a full stretch and a full contraction.

TRICEPS

FUNCTION #1: PRESSING MOVEMENTS

The elbow bends and straightens, and the upper arm simultaneously rotates up and down at the shoulder joint.

EXAMPLE EXERCISE

Bench Dip

STRETCH

The body is lowered, and the elbows are bent and rotated upward on a level with the shoulders.

CONTRACTION

The arms are straightened and the body's weight rests upon the flexed triceps.

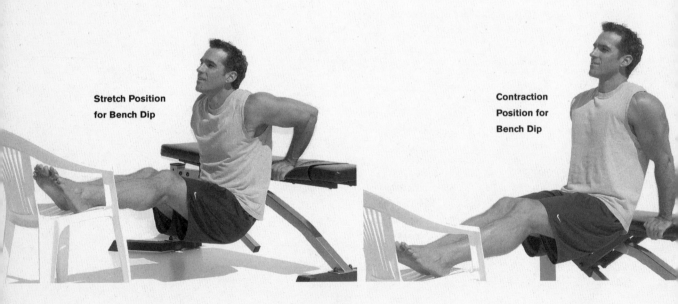

**Stretch Position
for Bench Dip**

**Contraction
Position for
Bench Dip**

Additional Triceps Pressing Movements

CLOSE-GRIP BENCH PRESSES

The hands are spaced about 12 inches apart on the bar, which is lowered to the bottom of the chest muscles for the stretch. The elbows should be kept close to the body (as opposed to straight out at a right angle from the torso, an angle that would target the chest).

MACHINE DIPS

The elbows should stay close to the body to emphasize the triceps.

FUNCTION #2: EXTENSION MOVEMENTS

The forearm is raised and lowered by a bending of the elbow. As opposed to the movement of the biceps curl, the force of effort is exerted through straightening the arm instead of bending it.

EXAMPLE EXERCISE

Lying Dumbbell Extension

STRETCH

The elbows are pointed toward the ceiling, with the hands next to the ears.

CONTRACTION

The arms are fully extended, with the elbows straightened and the dumbbells overhead. The flex should be focused away from the elbow joint and on the triceps muscle.

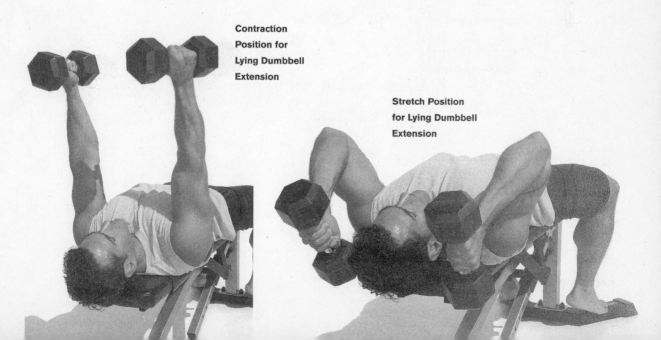

Contraction Position for Lying Dumbbell Extension

Stretch Position for Lying Dumbbell Extension

Additional Triceps Extension Movements

PUSH-DOWN

This is done by holding a short bar attached to a pulley machine. The stretch is reached by when, with the upper arms by the sides, the forearms are raised by bending the elbow until it touches the biceps. The contraction occurs when the bar is just in front of the thighs with the elbows straight and the triceps flexed.

BARBELL EXTENSION

This can be done either seated or lying down. Grip the bar (either a straight or curved curling bar) with the hands about 12 inches apart. Keep the elbows as close together as possible throughout the stretch and the contraction.

FOREARMS

FUNCTION #1: WRIST-CURLING MOVEMENTS

The wrist is bent and straightened by the forearm. Bending the palm inward flexes the under-forearm. Bending the back of the hand up flexes the top of the forearm.

EXAMPLE EXERCISE

Barbell Wrist Curl

STRETCH

The wrist is bent all the way back.

CONTRACTION

The wrist is bent forward so that the palm moves toward the flexed forearm.

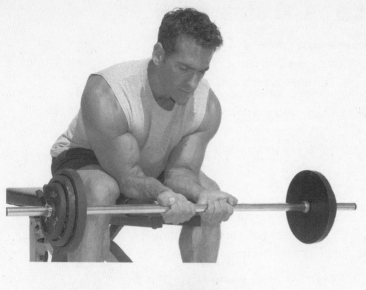

Stretch Position for Barbell Wrist Curl

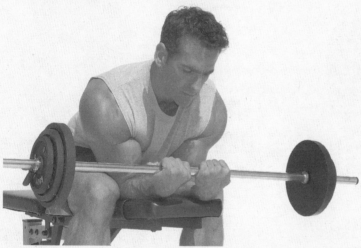

Contraction Position for Barbell Wrist Curl

Additional Wrist Curl Movement

DUMBBELL WRIST CURL

While standing, hold a dumbbell in each hand next to the thighs, and then curl and straighten the wrists.

PRIME

FRONT THIGHS

FUNCTION #1: EXTENSION MOVEMENTS

These are similar to a triceps-extension movement, with the knee acting as the elbow does there. The knee is bent and straightened.

EXAMPLE EXERCISE

Leg Extension

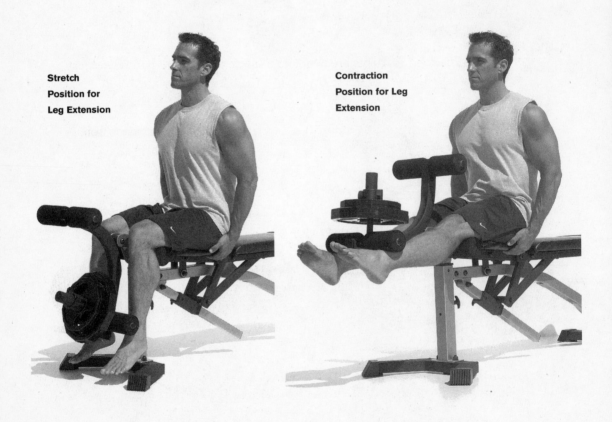

**Stretch
Position for
Leg Extension**

**Contraction
Position for Leg
Extension**

STRETCH

The knee is bent until the calf almost touches the back of the upper leg.

CONTRACTION

The knee is straightened with the front thigh muscles flexed.

FUNCTION #2: PRESSING MOVEMENTS

Like chest and shoulder pressing, these movements also involve two joints: in this case, the knee and the hip. The movement is similar to standing up from a chair.

EXAMPLE EXERCISE

Back Squats

STRETCH

The knee and hip joints are bent into a seated position, with the knees just past a 90-degree angle.

CONTRACTION

The knees and hips are straightened by standing up and flexing the front thighs.

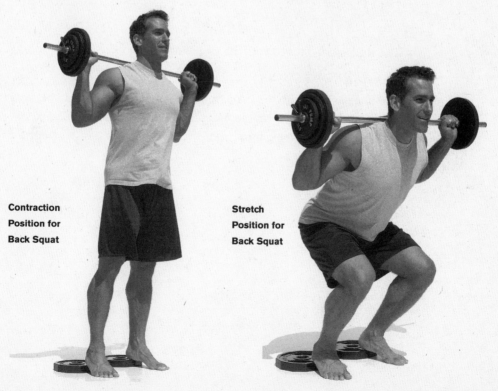

Contraction
Position for
Back Squat

Stretch
Position for
Back Squat

Additional Pressing Movements

LEG PRESS

This uses a machine that you sit in or lie on (depending on the style of equipment). The raising and lowering of the weight is done with a movement similar to the Squat.

HACK SQUAT

This is done on a machine that puts you into a more upright position. You then slide a weighted back rest up and down, duplicating the actions of a Back Squat.

HAMSTRINGS

FUNCTION #1: LEG CURL MOVEMENT

Similar to that of an arm biceps curl. The knee is bent until the calf touches the hamstrings.

EXAMPLE EXERCISE

Lying leg curl

STRETCH

The leg is straightened with the knee fully extended.

CONTRACTION

The knee is bent with the hamstrings flexed. The hips should be pushed down into the machine at the peak contraction of the movement, as opposed to letting the glutes rise up.

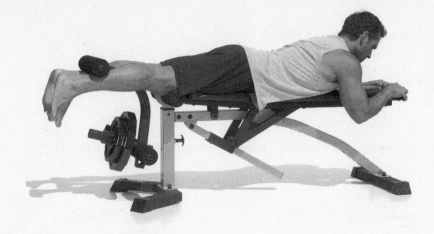

Stretch Position for Lying Leg Curl

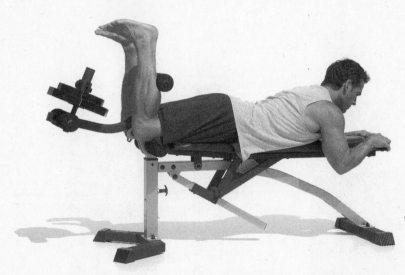

Contraction Position for Lying Leg Curl

Additional Hamstring Movement

STANDING LEG CURL

This is usually done on a machine that exercises one leg at a time.

FUNCTION #2

Stretching Movement

EXAMPLE EXERCISE

Good Mornings (see Back Function #3)

CALVES

FUNCTION #1: HEEL-RAISE MOVEMENTS

The heel is lowered and raised by extending the foot from the ankle.

EXAMPLE EXERCISE

Standing Calf Raise

STRETCHES

The heel is lowered from a raised block toward the ground by a bending of the ankle.

CONTRACTION

The heel is raised as high as possible by extending the foot from the ankle. The calf is flexed.

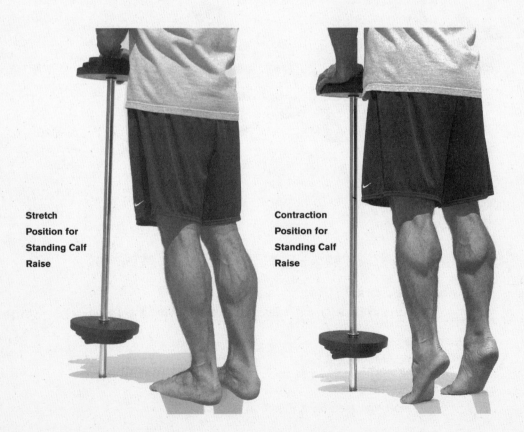

Stretch
Position for
Standing Calf
Raise

Contraction
Position for
Standing Calf
Raise

Additional Heel-Raise Movement

SEATED CALF RAISE

Using a machine on which you sit with a pad across your bent knees, the heels are raised and lowered against resistance.

ABDOMINALS

FUNCTION #1: CRUNCHING MOVEMENTS

The abdominal muscles (abs) are flexed by shortening the length of the area between the pelvis and the lower chest by curling the spine.

EXERCISE EXAMPLE

Crunch

STRETCH

With the upper body lying flat and the spine straight, the abdominals are lengthened.

CONTRACTION

The body is curled up, with the head in the direction of the knees; the abs are shortened and flexed.

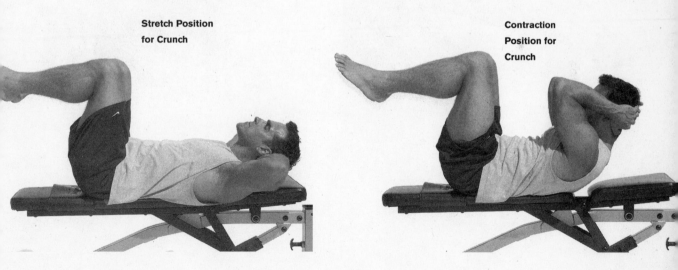

Stretch Position for Crunch

Contraction Position for Crunch

FUNCTION #2: LEG RAISE MOVEMENTS

The abs are shortened and lengthened by lifting the legs at the hip joint.

EXAMPLE EXERCISE

Lying Leg Raise

STRETCH

The legs are rotated at the hip joints down toward the ground.

CONTRACTION

The legs are raised; the pelvis is tilted upward; the abs are flexed.

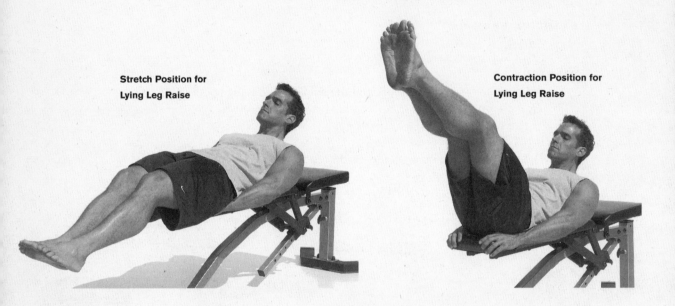

**Stretch Position for
Lying Leg Raise**

**Contraction Position for
Lying Leg Raise**

ISOMETRIC EXERCISES

In the *Prime* routines, I use five core isometric exercises. Each of these exercises concentrates on more than one key muscle group. When performing these exercises, you should use slow and sure movements. The key focus should be on the squeezing of the muscles.

Breathe as you exert the force, and inhale as you release. If it is a compound movement (like the Towel Pull-Down and Press), breathe out on each segment of the exertion and breathe in while holding the squeezed part of the movement. For example, on a Towel Pull-Down and Press, breathe out as you pull your arms down to flex the back, and while holding that flex, breathe in; as you push your arms back up (to flex the shoulders), breathe out; with arms extended and shoulders flexed, breathe in.

1.   CHEST PRESS
Primary stimulation: Chest

Bend at the elbows and bring the palms together close to the front of the chest. Press the hands together, flexing the chest muscles. Under control—and as if pushing against resistance—push the hands straight forward until the elbows are straightened. Squeeze the chest and bring the hands back toward the body.

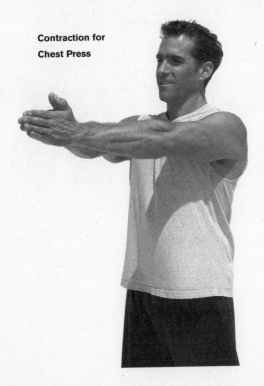

Contraction for
Chest Press

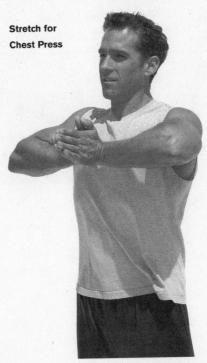

Stretch for
Chest Press

2. TOWEL PULL-DOWN AND PRESS
Primary stimulation: Back and Shoulders

With the arms overhead, grip a towel with your hands at shoulder width. Without moving the hands on the towel, push them outward, exerting tension. Now, by bending the elbows, pull the hands downward, squeezing the back muscles (as in a pull-down weight exercise). Hold the squeeze, and then, keeping the tension of the hands pushing outward, use the shoulder muscles to slowly press the hands back up until the elbows are straight.

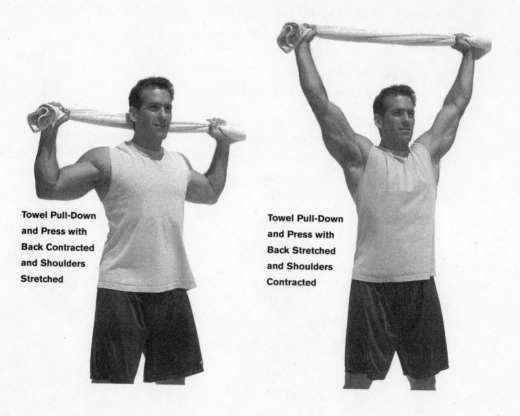

Towel Pull-Down and Press with Back Contracted and Shoulders Stretched

Towel Pull-Down and Press with Back Stretched and Shoulders Contracted

3. LEG PRESS AND ROW:
Primary stimulation: Back and Thighs

Lying on the floor with your legs bent, hook a towel over the feet, holding on to each end with your hands. As you straighten your legs, flex them, but also give resistance with your back muscles, as if stretching in a rowing exercise. When your knees are straightened, flex the legs, and then begin to pull against the leg resistance with the back muscles, as if you're pulling something toward your ribcage. Flex the back as the elbows bend.

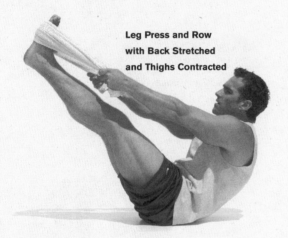

**Leg Press and Row
with Back Stretched
and Thighs Contracted**

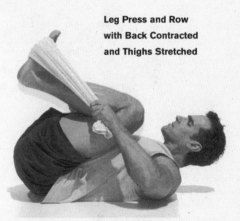

**Leg Press and Row
with Back Contracted
and Thighs Stretched**

4. BALLET SQUAT
Primary stimulation: Thighs and Glutes (butt muscles)

With feet spread at shoulder width and toes pointed outward, squeeze the glutes and bend at the knees, as if beginning to sit in a chair. Stop about a quarter of the way down and flex the thighs and butt. Hold the position, and then straighten the legs again.

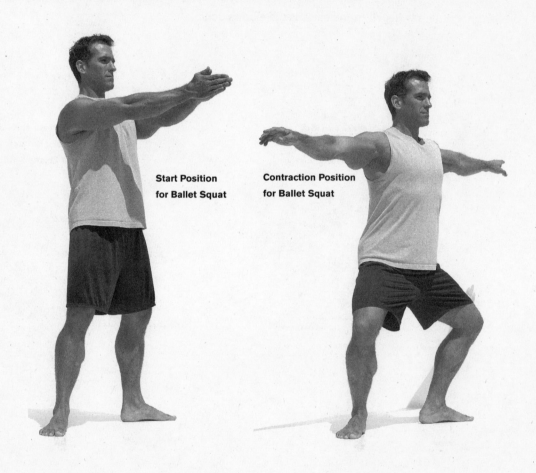

**Start Position
for Ballet Squat**

**Contraction Position
for Ballet Squat**

5. TOWEL SIDE RAISE
Primary stimulation: Shoulders

With a towel held in both hands, extend one slightly bent arm outward and up to the side, flexing the shoulder muscles. Provide resistance with the opposite arm. When one hand is parallel to the ground, hold the flex of the shoulder and then allow the other arm to pull—against the opposite arm's resistance—downward in front of the body until it too is raised. The repetitions will be done as if see-sawing back and forth under complete control.

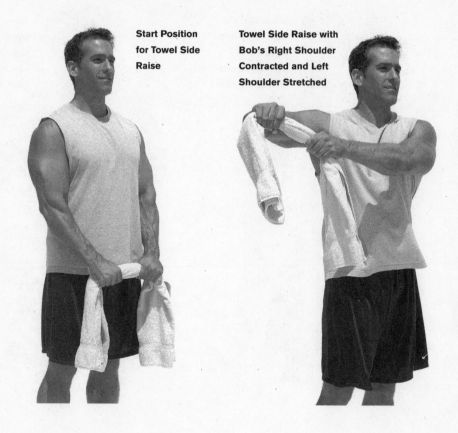

Start Position for Towel Side Raise

Towel Side Raise with Bob's Right Shoulder Contracted and Left Shoulder Stretched

6. TOWEL CURL AND PUSHDOWN
Primary stimulation: Biceps and Triceps

Holding a towel with your hands close together and one palm facing up and the other down, bend the elbow of the palm-up hand until the biceps are flexed. Resist with the other arm all the way up. Then, with that other arm, push down against the curled arm, using it as resistance, and flex the triceps. Switch arms after the prescribed number of reps.

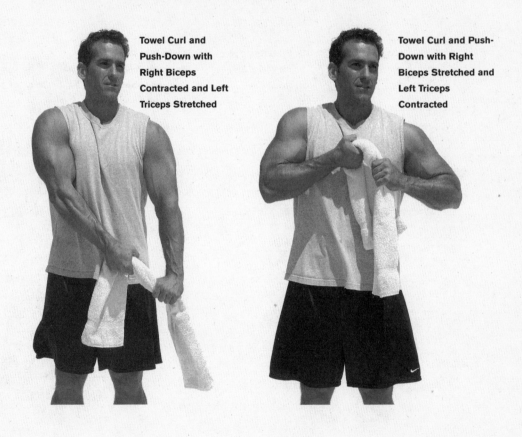

Towel Curl and Push-Down with Right Biceps Contracted and Left Triceps Stretched

Towel Curl and Push-Down with Right Biceps Stretched and Left Triceps Contracted

STRENGTHEN YOUR HEART AND LUNGS

Two of the most important fitness and health issues facing the 40+ man are his cardiovascular health and his endurance levels. In addition to building strength in the muscular system, every man should do exercises that target the health of his heart and lungs. To do this requires a slightly different form of exercise than the resistance training described earlier.

Resistance training strengthens the skeletal muscles and the connective tissues, and yet it only has a small amount of impact on cardiovascular fitness and endurance.

In order to exercise and strengthen the heart and lungs—which has the added benefit of stoking the metabolism and thus helping the body to burn calories more efficiently—you must elevate the heart rate within a target range and maintain it there consistently for a certain amount of time.

Cardiovascular training (cardio) differs from resistance training in both style of exercise and intensity. With resistance training, a high intensity-level is desirable for producing superior results. With cardio training, a moderate intensity-level is most desirable; you strive essentially to lose your breath to a certain level and maintain that state for a minimum of 12 minutes (the minimum amount of time needed to derive cardiovascular benefit) and up to an hour. When you get your pulse elevated and your lungs activated and maintain that condition for a while, you strengthen your heart muscles and raise the endurance levels of your body. This increase in specific strength definitely compliments the strengths built through resistance workouts. The wonderful thing about both resistance training and cardiovascular workouts is that they have a combined (and essentially synergistic) positive impact on a man's body and health.

Since a portion of the benefit that comes from a properly targeted cardio workout is directed toward the metabolism—and therefore toward fat-burning—you want to plan the intensity of your workout to maximize the outcome. The beauty of a properly performed cardio workout is that it doesn't just burn calories and fat during the workout; it also boosts the metabolic rate for up to four hours afterward. Can you see the amazing benefits of doing that?

You can't approach a cardio exercise as if you're trying to do an all-out, gut-busting weight exercise. You aren't trying to stimulate your outer muscles through high intensity. In other words, if you're doing a cardio exercise and it's making the muscles of your legs burn like a Leg Press set might, you're working too hard. You may have the setting too high (the tension setting on a stationary bike, or the hill-incline angle on a treadmill, for example), or you may be moving too fast. The goal is to raise the pulse into a target range, not to over-stimulate skeletal muscles. In fact, the muscles that you want to work are inside your chest; the heart and the muscles around the lungs are stimulated differently than are the skeletal muscles. Also the exercise that you do for cardio shouldn't be thought of as if you're in a race. It's simply the means of stimulating a particular positive response from the heart and lungs (and, as a bonus, the metabolism).

So how do you maximize the benefits of cardio training? The basics are simple. Pick an exercise (I'll list my favorites for the 40+ man in a moment) that will get your heart rate into the target range, and keep up that activity at a steady pace for as much time as you want to keep going. Generally, this is between 12 and 30 minutes, depending on the exercise, intensity, experience and conditioning levels, and desired goal.

What is a target heart rate? A simple formula can provide your target heart-rate range, which will be personalized according to your age and desired intensity. Your target heart rate can be calculated by subtracting your age from the number 220 and then multiplying that number by a percentage between 60 and 70 percent.

The percentage represents the intensity of the exercise measured by heartbeats per minute. One hundred percent would be your all-out heart rate capacity, which would be nearly impossible (not to mention undesirable) to sustain for any length of time. The middle-ground meeting point between an intensity that will provide cardio fitness and a level that will burn fat rather than muscle glycogen (undesirable for fat loss) is in the range between 60 and 70 percent. You should target 70 percent if your cardio workout is in the 12-to-30 minute range and 60 percent if it is longer.

So let's look at this calculation for a moment. If you're 40 years old and want to work-out in the 60-percent range, your heart-rate calculation would be:

$$220 - 40 = 180$$
$$180 \times .60 = 108$$

Therefore, your target heart-rate range, which you would strive to maintain throughout the cardio exercise, would be 108 beats per minute. At 70 percent, it would be 116 beats per minute.

You can take your pulse very quickly by placing the first two fingers of one hand on the inside of your wrist, just under the thumb joint of the other hand, and timing your pulse for six seconds, then adding a zero on the end of that. (Let's say the six-second pulse is 12 beats; add a zero, that's 120 beats per minute—just slightly over the target range, but acceptable.)

A good rule of thumb with heart-rate level during cardio workouts is that you should be able to carry on a conversation (even if it's a bit winded-sounding) while in your target range. As you might expect, that doesn't mean that I suggest it. I like to do affirmations and positive visualization during my cardio workouts, and I believe that it's of far greater benefit to my overall fitness and wellness goals than it is to chat about the weather with the guy on the next treadmill.

I can't overemphasize how important it is for the 40+ man to dedicate time and energy to some form of cardio training.

THE BEST CARDIO EXERCISES FOR THE 40+ MAN

An essential aspect of effective cardio exercise is that it enables a man to get his pulse rate into the target range, yet not be overly jarring on the joints, ligaments, and bones. Many men assume that if they want to get their hearts in shape, they should simply lace up the running shoes and set out on a five-mile jog. This isn't the best strategy, for a couple of reasons. The first is that by the time the average man reaches 40—and especially if he's been inactive for a while—his knees, feet, and lower back aren't going to be able to take the pounding of a run. The second reason is simply that, for most men, running elevates the heart-rate above the target zone. As I said earlier, one of the benefits of working in the 60- to 70-percent zone is that fat is used for the majority of the fuel during the workout. Again, you seek only a certain level of intensity to meet the blended, maximized levels of cardio and endurance conditioning, metabolic boost, and fat loss. It is vastly superior for the goals of the *Prime* program to do cardio for a longer time at a lower intensity than to put in a brief, all-out burst.

It is also important to note that the time when cardio exercise is performed will affect how efficiently the target heart-rate range is reached and maintained. In many of the *Prime* routines, I will suggest blending cardio work with resistance and flexibility workouts. Usually, cardio will follow resistance training. The reasons are simple:

- If you begin a cardio exercise cold, it may take up to several minutes just to get the pulse rate into the target zone.

- If you follow your resistance workout with cardio, your pulse rate will already be elevated from the other exercise, and all you'll have to do is keep it there. This makes the time spent on cardio more efficient (since you'll be spending the entire workout in the target zone), and you'll already have the body warmed up.

This doesn't mean that there isn't value in doing a cardio exercise on its own. It simply means that if you do, you'll need to allow time for the pulse rate to get into the zone.

It's interesting to observe—as something of a related side-note—that the average man spends about 95 percent of his time indoors. Don't limit your active life to just the structured exercises in this book. *Prime* is also a call to get active in your own life. Get outside. Plant a garden. Go to the woods or a park. Swim in a lake. Play golf or tennis, or roll around in the grass with your kids or your dog. Whatever you do, use the conditioning that you get from your structured workouts to motivate you to get out from in front of the TV and get active.

There are any number of different exercises that can be used for cardio workouts—so long as the activity:

1. Is steady; doesn't require constant starting and stopping;

2. Is performed at moderate intensity;

3. Keeps the heart rate in the target range.

My three favorites are:

■ Cycling, either on a stationary bike or outdoors. You should make sure that you're spinning the pedals at a low-tension setting, using high revolutions per minute to avoid creating too much muscle burn in the thighs (as opposed to a high-tension and low RPMs). If you cycle outdoors, you must find a way to keep moving. I'm not saying that simply going out and riding a bike isn't valuable. I often use my bike as a means of transportation and recreation. It's simply that, as a goal-oriented cardio workout, the exercise must be steady. Stop-and-go traffic prevents this. That's why I recommend that you cycle outdoors for recreation and use a stationary bike for cardio workouts. Also, make sure that your seat height is properly adjusted. On an indoor or an outdoor bike, your knees should go to about a 97-percent lock-out when the pedal is at its farthest point of extension.

■ Stair Climbing Machine: Again, the tension on the machine should be moderate, and the actual step speed (the rate at which you step up and down) should be fast (yet controlled). The major caution here is that this exercise, unless done with complete attention to form, is hard on many men's knees. To counteract this (unless you have a knee injury that precludes the exercise altogether), you should keep each step smooth and gliding, with no joint-snapping or bouncing at the top or bottom. Try to find a normal step range, somewhere between the knees-barely-bending waddle that you see some people use and the knees-up-to-the-chest technique of others. Stay smooth and steady. You can also do stair-climbing without a machine, but you'd need either a very tall building with staircase access or a long, steep flight of outdoor steps.

■ Power Walking: This is far and away my favorite way to get my cardio workout, simply because it's the safest (in terms of injury prevention) and the most enjoyable. I've been known to use an indoor treadmill for this, but I usually get outdoors. I'm fortunate to live near trails and natural areas, but even in the city, I simply love to walk. I don't mean stroll along and window shop, or stop to look at the view every couple of minutes. I'm talking about purposeful striding, taking long powerful steps, using the arms and moving fast. Power walking is superior to running for fat burning. An all-out run might burn between 800 and 1,000 calories per hour, but only a highly trained athlete can run at that pace (most men would collapse and likely get injured). Walking at a rapid pace may burn only between 500 and 600 calories per hour, but the goal is also to use body fat as the main fuel source. The run would only use about five percent body fat as fuel (because of intensity), whereas the power walk would shift that percentage of fat calories burned to around 60 percent. This is much more efficient, not to mention the fact that the walk is far more body-friendly and allows you to exercise longer and therefore get the heart into better and better shape. You can also perform a variation of this exercise by marching in place. I use this in some of the upcoming routines.

BUILD FLEXIBILITY

I don't particularly care for sweeping generalizations, but I'll offer one here: In general, men hate to stretch. Even men who are experienced with exercise rarely stretch their bodies, and when they do, it's usually a few seconds of bounce-and-be-done-with-it, after which they move along to something more "productive." Yet there's growing and powerful evidence showing that when a man changes his lifestyle to improve his overall health, relaxation and flexibility play roles every bit as essential as do muscle strength and proper nutrition. There's a synergistic cooperation in which properly performed and directed stretching (especially when blended with the relaxation techniques discussed in MOTIVATED MIND) becomes a cornerstone of a man's overall wellness.

Let me be absolutely clear: Flexibility is an essential portion of building a fit body—

PRIME

every bit as important as strength and cardio training. If you don't have a high level of flexibility, your efforts in the gym will be decreased and your body will age much more rapidly.

The underactive 40+ man isn't just losing muscle and gaining fat; he's also becoming far less flexible with each passing year, and this will have adverse effects on his health, quality of life, and self-image. What good does it do to be physically fit if you can't even bend over and touch your toes, or can't get your hand around behind you to scratch your back?

Many of what we consider to be our injuries—and certainly our physical tight spots—are directly related to a lack of muscular flexibility. In order to achieve true levels of fitness, it's necessary to adopt a systematic approach to stretching.

While resistance training involves a certain amount of stretching, it is mainly a muscle-tensing activity. You're essentially clenching your muscles against resistance. I want you to see the flexibility exercises described below as a way to work against a different kind of resistance. That resistance is the tension that builds up in the body not just during weight-training exercise or inactivity, but also through the physical and mental efforts of working against gravity day after day—the physical gravity that pulls on the body and the other kinds that pull at the spirit. Stretching is a release from that tension; a way to loosen the muscles and the mind. Because we live in a world that produces stress at so many levels, your stretching routines will be a key route to both flexibility and relaxation. Those are the two major benefits of stretching: You must relax into the movements in order to become more physically flexible, and you will thus become more relaxed as flexibility increases.

Think of your body (especially those tight muscles) as rubber bands on a cold morning. If you take a rubber band outside in the cold and pull it tight, it will likely break. If you slowly stretch it out a bit at a time, with patience, it will become as if alive; it will be pliable and completely useful.

Think of stretching as lengthening the muscles. You should go into a stretch slowly and hold it, while breathing in a relaxed way. Every stretch should be held for at least 20 seconds without bouncing or over-forcing the muscles. Don't make it about trying to be the most flexible man in the room. As with weight training, in which you should set your ego aside and not try to compete with others, with stretching you should also release all sense of competitiveness.

I see stretching as serving some very important functions in a well-rounded fitness lifestyle. These things become incredibly important to the 40+ man, who will be amazed as he becomes limber and relaxed, integrating his resistance exercise, cardio workouts, and flexibility training into a balanced program.

Stretching is:

- An aid to injury rehabilitation

- A relaxation exercise

- A means to attain a peaceful outlook

- A self-contained program for better mobility

- An exercise warmup

- A cooldown after exercise

- An aid in falling asleep

- An aid in waking up

- An adjunct to help vitalize growth in stubborn body parts

In fact, stretching is so important to the 40+ man that if I were forced to make a single choice between weights, cardio, and proper stretching, I would have to choose stretching. Without mobility, you cannot move freely, and the quality of life is impacted. I cannot imagine slowly growing stiffer and less mobile with age, without any physical disability, simply because I'd refused to take the time to do something that's so clearly good for me.

I use what I call Power Stretching in my own life and in the *Prime* routines. Power Stretching draws on both more traditional athletic stretches and some aspects of yoga.

While yoga has become much more popular in recent years for a number of extraordinarily powerful reasons, *Prime* is not a book about yoga. I simply draw some of the positive benefits from this four-thousand-year-old tradition, which is known to harness the power of the body and mind, helping one—among other things—relax and come alive. Yoga blends aspects of exercise with elements of meditation and proper breathing and an attentiveness that I find absolutely compelling. Yoga was first considered a pathway to healing that helped unify the body and mind, leading to a sense of peace and enlightenment. Many of its aspects act as a gentle method of putting the overstressed body back into a state of interior and exterior wellness.

That said, I merely incorporate elements which I consider to be yoga-like (including the use of some basic yoga movements and names for a few of the stretches) in my Power Stretching exercises, which will, in turn, be integrated into the *Prime* routines.

THE POWER STRETCHES

CHEST AND BICEPS STRETCH

Depending on hand placement, this can emphasize either chest or biceps in the stretch. Place one hand against a stationary object at head height and slowly rotate the body away from the supported, outstretched arm, opening up the chest. To emphasize the chest, point the palm forward; for biceps, the palm faces toward the ground.

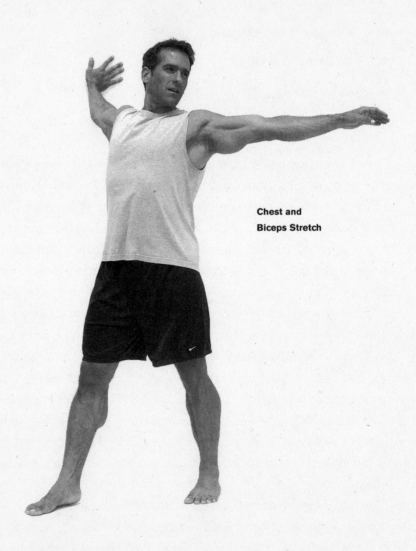

**Chest and
Biceps Stretch**

BACK AND HAMSTRING STRETCH

Bend slowly from the waist and, with one hand, grab the opposite ankle. If flexibility is a problem, bend at the knees. Straighten the knees slightly to intensify the stretch, and gently pull against the ankle, finding the back stretch. Be careful with the lower back in this position.

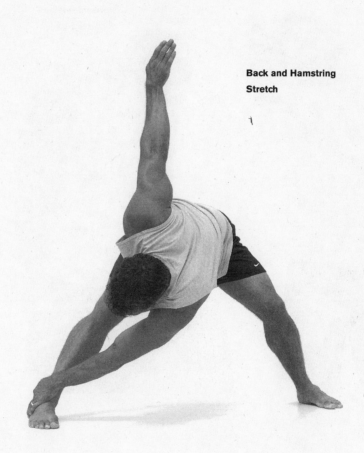

Back and Hamstring Stretch

NECK ROLL

Standing upright, first gently roll the head forward, pushing the chin as far down toward the chest as possible. Then roll the head straight back until you're looking up at the ceiling. Bring the head back to normal and stretch to one side, gently assisting with the arm over the head, and then roll the head to the other side.

Side Position for Neck Roll

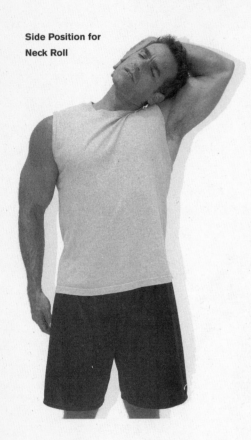

Forward Position for Neck Roll

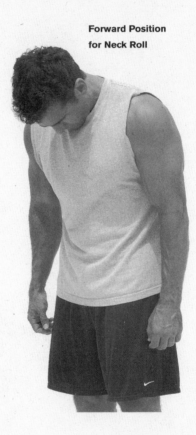

Back Position for Neck Roll

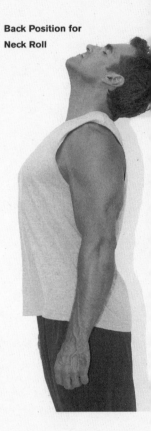

SHOULDER AND TRICEPS STRETCH

This creates shoulder mobility and triceps flexibility. Holding a towel (or belt) in one hand and lowering it over the same side's shoulder, grab the towel with the other hand behind the back. Slowly and gently, continue to "climb" the behind-the-back hand up the towel, edging it closer to the top hand. Watch those shoulder joints—they can be quite fragile.

Shoulder and Triceps Stretch

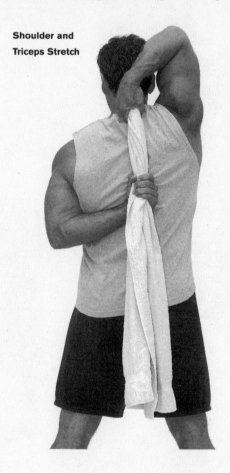

PRIME

137 GATHER THE FACTS

FORWARD BEND

With the feet shoulder-width apart, put the arms above the head and gently roll the spine forward. At first, keep the knees bent. Roll the upper body as far forward as possible, and hang. Try straightening the knees a bit, if it's physically possible. Bend the knees slightly to accommodate rolling the spine back upward until you're standing up straight again.

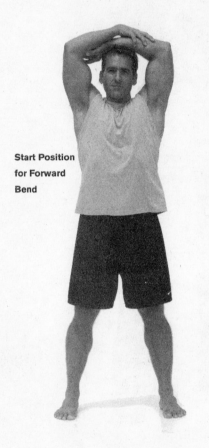

Start Position for Forward Bend

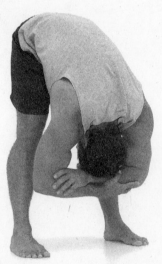

Forward Bend

WARRIOR I

This works to restore the spine's flexibility and can be good for upper back and neck stiffness. Begin in a wide stance with the hands out to the sides. Bring the hands together directly overhead with the arms straight. Turn on the right foot until the trunk (upper body) is facing right. Stretch back to the left heel, bending at the knee of the right leg. Lift the hands and upper body toward the ceiling and look up at the hands. Hold the pose for the prescribed length of time. Breathe in deeply and reverse the process. Then repeat on the other side.

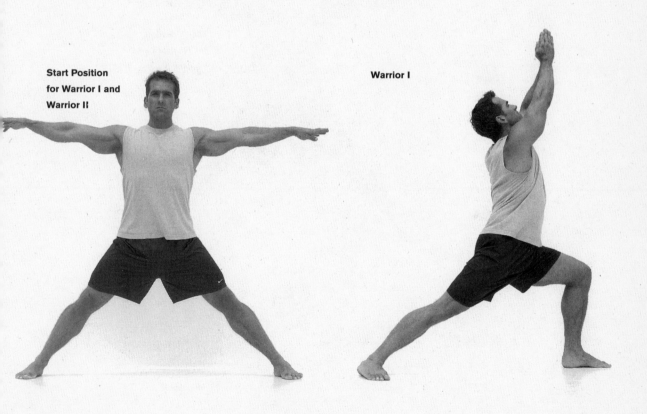

Start Position for Warrior I and Warrior II

Warrior I

WARRIOR II

This helps develop the thighs and calves. Begin in the same position as for Warrior I. Feet should be parallel and about four feet apart. Rotate the left foot slightly inward and the right foot all the way outward. Rotate the upper body from the waist and bend into the leg, in the direction in which you are rotating. Keep the arms in a straight line and look in the direction of the bent knee. Breathe deeply, hold the pose, reverse the process, and then repeat on the opposite side.

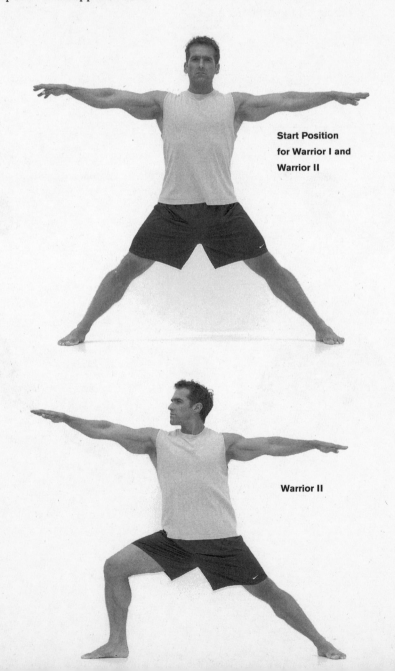

**Start Position
for Warrior I and
Warrior II**

Warrior II

WIDE LEG STRETCH

This one is for hips, thighs, and lower back. From the wide stance (as in the Warrior poses), put the hands on the hips and gain balance, then roll forward with the upper body and place the hands on the floor even with the feet and shoulder-width apart. Stretch the spine forward and, bending at the elbows, take the head to the floor. Hold the stretch, and then reverse the process to stand up.

Wide Leg Stretch

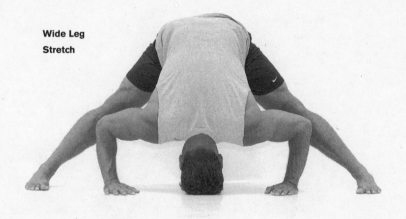

HEAD TO KNEE STRETCH

This structure is for the hips, lower back, and hamstrings. Sitting on the ground with one leg extended, bend the other leg at the knee until the foot is against the opposite inner thigh. Roll forward with the spine and take the head toward the extended knee. Grab the foot to assist with the tension. Breathe and relax. Hold the stretch, then roll back up and repeat on the opposite side.

Head-to-Knee Stretch

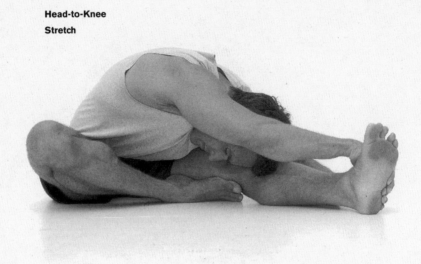

TWIST

This one is for spinal flexibility. Sitting upright in a cross-legged position, rotate the upper body to one side and then to the other. Hold each stretch, and use the hands to extend the range of motion. Be sure to lift up with the upper body as you twist and to keep the posture completely upright.

Start Position for Twist

Twist

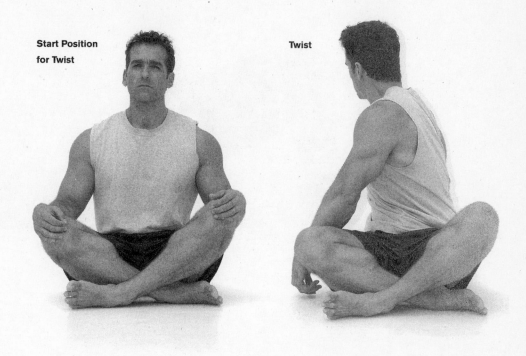

BRIDGE

Good for stretching and strengthening the back. Lie with the feet hip-width apart and the arms extended along the sides. Pull the heels up toward the butt. Reach the hands toward the heels and raise the hips as high into the air as possible, pushing the feet down against the floor. You can lift up on the balls of the feet to further extend the stretch.

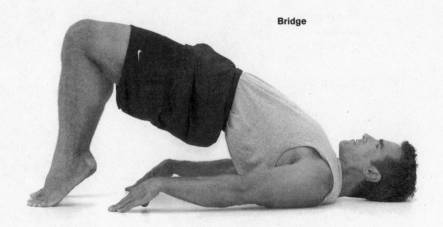

Bridge

LOCUST

Great for strengthening and stretching the muscles around the spine. Lying on the stomach with the arms extended along the sides, the chin up, and the legs together, simply raise the head and the feet simultaneously. Try to get the arms up level with the shoulder joints. Look forward as you hold the stretch, and breathe.

Locust

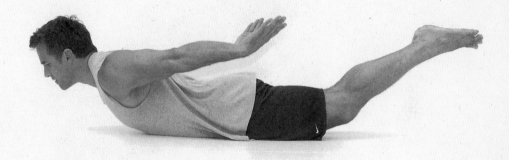

CAMEL

This is great for correcting "desk posture"—the rolled-forward slump. While on your knees and with the hips pushed forward and centered under the spine, breathe out and allow the head to fall back. Reach the hands straight behind you and try to touch the ankles. Take this slowly. Hold the maximum individual stretch, and then roll back forward, breathing deeply.

Camel

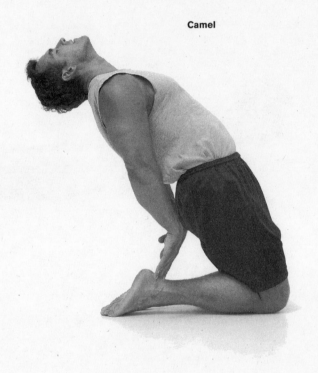

CREATE ROUTINES

I wrote this book for men who want to revolutionize their fitness lives. There are many ways to go about creating that revolution. The first is for the man to begin moving again—to take action on his own behalf to improve his overall health and fitness levels. The other is to explore training methods that fall outside the more traditional ways of working out. Most books like this would now give one or two simple weight-training workouts, with some cardio and stretching advice tacked on (almost as an afterthought). I have never taken that approach.

I believe that if you're going to revolutionize your fitness life, you must really seek an entirely new way of doing things. That doesn't mean that traditional knowledge won't be utilized, but revolutionary workouts turn the traditions inside-out and establish new, bold ways to get the job done.

To create a *Prime* body, you must go beyond the simplistic exercise routines that have become almost like a dogmatic, worn-out mantra in the fitness industry. That's what I seek to provide: a step beyond the ordinary (although I should note here that I do also include some traditional weight-training routines for those who seek that information).

When I began exercising again after having left the intense training of competition behind, I knew that I didn't want to use my old style of working out, which, while certainly effective for bodybuilding, wasn't a perfect method for creating the new style of body that I was seeking. I didn't want massive bulk; I wanted to be sleek and muscular; strong, flexible, and totally fit. I wanted workouts that would begin to compensate for the changes that were taking place as I left my mid-30s behind. I needed ways of training that would counteract the natural decline in my body's own production of the hormones that keep younger men lean and muscular. I wanted something brand new. But, even in approaching some new methods, I still looked to the elements that I'd always used to create results-oriented training routines. I knew that every workout needed to be:

BALANCED

Any ideal workout should be balanced in all of its elements. For example, training should seek a balance between strength, flexibility, and endurance. Therefore, every program should take these into account. There should also be a balance between the various body parts. Each muscle group is important. I don't subscribe to the school of thought that says that you should only build the "showy" muscles, like the chest and biceps. This leads to a very unbalanced look, and it doesn't respect the wholeness of a synergistic system. Muscles work together. They are cooperative (like the way the chest, shoulders, and triceps work in conjunction in some movements, for example) and also oppose each other. For example, the chest and the back are opposing body parts, as are the biceps and triceps, and the front thighs and hamstrings. The opposition of these muscle groups is what enables the body to move, so it is essential that muscles on each side of these oppositions be treated equally in any workout routine.

Also, there must be a balance between the elements of stimulation and recuperation. This is best expressed by creating a balance between workout duration and available rest time. All of the *Prime* routines will take these various elements of balance into consideration.

STRUCTURED

Without a structured organization of body parts, exercises, sets, and repetitions, a workout would be a state of chaos from which only minor progress would be possible. Workouts are formally structured so that the experience can be observed and understood. If you simply went to the gym and wandered around doing a few reps of this thing, then a few reps of something else, without consideration of structure, you'd get nowhere. It would be like trying to get to New York by wandering aimlessly around a few California back roads. Each of the *Prime* routines will be carefully structured, so that you can understand whether or not it is working for you and can adapt accordingly.

GOAL-FOCUSED

You should always know what to expect—what you are working toward—in any exercise program. If you go into a gym with the notion of building a sleek, lean body but train like a power-lifter, your goal and your work won't mesh. As you enter into a program, you should have some reasonable idea of where that program will take you. I've included a wide variety of workout programs that are tailored to a variety of goals—from attaining greater flexibility to building muscle mass.

The *Prime* routines are made up of different styles of training, each of which is balanced, structured, and focused on a particular fitness goal.

POWER FLEX

This is a blending of elements of the yoga-like stretches with the other flexibility exercises, combined with some very focused isometrics and light-weight (but high-intensity) resistance exercises, and it emphasizes every body part. The core goal of a Power Flex workout isn't building muscle mass so much as lengthening and toning the muscles while creating a tremendous increase in flexibility.

MUSCLE BLAST

This is a brief, intense workout designed for the man who wants to maximize the subtle triggering of the body's growth hormone releases (which decline with age, but are stimulated by brief, intense resistance exercise). Compound exercises, which stimulate the synergistic muscle systems in minimal time, are blended with intense stretches and isometrics.

NATURAL BODY BUILDER

This is an approach toward training for the man who wants to add muscle mass to his body. The workouts are designed to allow for the optimal amount of recuperation time and will also emphasize flexibility and cardio work.

Of course, each of the various routines is specifically designed to take into account the stimulation and recuperation needs of the 40+ man. There will also be a section of Basic Flexibility and Isometric Sequences. These are designed as warmup routines, but they can be used on their own as well as a means of developing greater flexibility.

There are some important points to consider as you enter into a *Prime* program:

1. Respect your experience level. If you're an absolute beginner, don't try to do advanced workouts. That's counterproductive. It does you no good to be gung-ho for one or two workouts, get extremely sore, and quit.

2. Always warm up and cool down whenever you train. You must respect the machinery of your body.

3. If you ever feel dizzy or sick during a workout, sit down and rest. If, once you've caught your breath, you feel able to continue, go slowly.

4. Stay focused on what you're doing at all times. See your physical exercises as strengthening the body and the mind.

5. Pay attention to the signals that your body is sending you. Learn the difference between muscle burn and injury before it's too late.

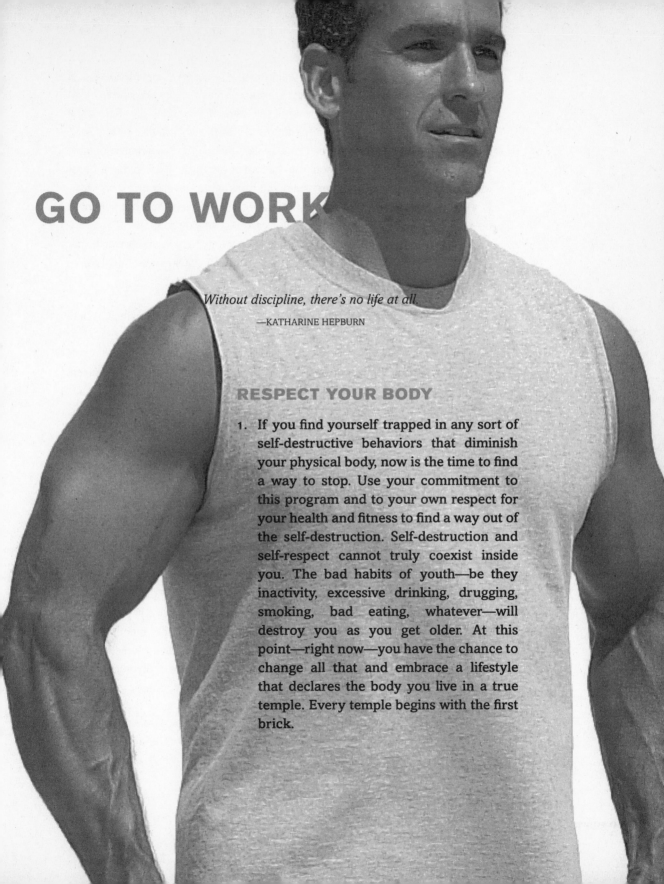

GO TO WORK

Without discipline, there's no life at all.
—KATHARINE HEPBURN

RESPECT YOUR BODY

1. If you find yourself trapped in any sort of self-destructive behaviors that diminish your physical body, now is the time to find a way to stop. Use your commitment to this program and to your own respect for your health and fitness to find a way out of the self-destruction. Self-destruction and self-respect cannot truly coexist inside you. The bad habits of youth—be they inactivity, excessive drinking, drugging, smoking, bad eating, whatever—will destroy you as you get older. At this point—right now—you have the chance to change all that and embrace a lifestyle that declares the body you live in a true temple. Every temple begins with the first brick.

2.   If you've been inactive for several years or if you haven't ever taken care of your health and fitness, declare a new start for yourself. Truly tell yourself that 40 (or whatever your current age is) is the start of your new life. Reject the notion that many sedentary men tell themselves: *My body will take care of itself.* Nonsense. Right now, as you read this, realize that if you take charge of how you treat your body, you can keep from becoming seriously ill down the not-too-distant road. Taking charge won't keep you from aging—everyone grows older. It will, however, change the quality of your aging process. Ask yourself right now if you would rather make a small investment in exercise (few of the routines in this book take longer than 45 minutes a day); if you aren't worth that effort. Get off the couch. Turn off the television. Take care of that body you're living in.

3.   We live in a culture in which it has become very fashionable to be cynical. While this is sometimes just a biting perspective on the world we live in, a cynical or negative attitude toward self-care is especially defeating for anyone who needs to make a positive change. Reject all notions of cynicism regarding how you feel about and treat your body. You've reached an age at which you have a choice between allowing yourself to decline or embrace positive change. If the whole idea of positive change, good body-image, and other aspects of self-care bring out a nasty streak, be willing to take a step back and try to find out if your negativity is a defense mechanism. Sometimes we become nasty about what consistently feels unattainable. I'm here to tell you that no matter where you are right now, you can create positive change in your life, and that change will be self-perpetuating. There is no more effective tool against the downward spiral of self-directed negativity than making some forward progress with your fitness and wellness goals.

4.   Using the visualization skills discussed in MOTIVATED MIND, sit down, relax, and imagine your own body, picturing what you would feel like if you were to turn yourself and your body into a fit and healthy machine, functioning on every level; moving freely, sexually active, strong and alive. See yourself in situations that make you feel great about this body that you're imagining. Do this every day, and allow this image to evolve as you invest in your new routine.

5.   Using your journal, sit down in a relaxed and private place. Draw a line down the middle of a blank journal page from top to bottom. On the top of the left-hand column, write STRENGTHS, and on top of the right-hand column, write

WEAKNESSES. We're going to do the first part of an honest analysis of where your body is right now in terms of shape and fitness. Think about your body as it is right now. Then add a twist: Use your imagination to see yourself from another person's perspective. Imagine that you're someone else who happens to care about *you* very much, who will tell you the truth without being too gentle or too harsh. Let this imaginary person write on your journal page what your body's physical strengths and weaknesses are. Give yourself about five minutes to do this exercise. It can be a first step in helping you analyze your body from the relative safety of an imaginary distance.

6.   Now I want you to take an honest look in the mirror and make your own analysis. The only way to know how to proceed with your workouts is to know what needs work. To do that, you have to become familiar with your own body. Are you the sort of man who has allowed himself to get so out-of-shape that you won't look at yourself in a full-length mirror naked? I'd like you to change that today. Turn the page in your journal and create another pair of STRENGTH and WEAKNESS columns. Go to a private full-length mirror and take off all your clothes. Even if you aren't shy, I want you to do this exercise completely alone. There should be no other opinions in the room. Now take a look at yourself with honest eyes. Don't beat up on yourself or cut yourself too much slack. Stand up straight, but don't suck your gut in or flex; be natural. How do you honestly feel that you look? What sort of shape are you in? What are the parts of your body that you like and the parts that you hate? Examine your body from the front and sides. Head to toe. Get a mirror so that you can look from the back. Write in your journal what you feel your strengths and weaknesses are as you stand there today. Be totally honest. Remember that your journal is for your eyes only, and that you shouldn't hold back in this kind of personal exercise.

7.   With the two lists you've made—one from an imaginary outside perspective and one from yours—begin to establish a firm idea of which physical areas you need to work on. You will structure your exercise routines based in part on this information. Do you feel that you have more weaknesses than strengths? Don't let that get you down. Certainly don't allow it to keep you from moving forward. My philosophy has always been that when we exercise, we shouldn't just work on the areas that are our strengths. We should fall in love with our weaknesses. In other words, when you get to your exercise routines, don't simply focus on the muscle groups that are strong in your body. Train them, yes, but also learn to love the weak body parts. They are the ones that need the most attention,

after all. If you have a strong chest but weak legs, your legs should get your attention. If you feel that body fat is a weakness, make reducing it a top priority, rather than just focusing on—for example—building a muscle that responds easily to training. I believe that not only will you build a more balanced-looking body, but that it is through working on our weaknesses in life (with our bodies and otherwise) that we best grow. Weaknesses present us with frustrations to break through; they give us the gift of making us pay attention and develop better strategies to change them. This is once again a return to that all-important concept of *attention* being the best road to improvement.

DEVELOP MUSCLE

1. When doing any type of resistance workout, always warm up the muscle first by performing a much lighter, less-intense set of the exercise. Never launch into an intense weight-training workout without doing this. If you imagine that your muscles are like rubber bands on a cold day, then you know that to keep them from "snapping," you must stretch them out a bit at a time, slowly. Each workout will have a warming-up aspect that should not be ignored. Perhaps a man can get away with skipping his warmups when he is very young, but with age, the muscles and all of the connective tissues lose elasticity and require being treated with respect.

2. If you have never done an exercise before, perform what I call a "rehearsal." Take a very, very light weight and perform the exercise, trying to find the perfect form: the stretch, the contraction, the perfect, sweet pathway between the two. You can also use this as something of a warmup. Begin by doing the movement without intensity and, with each progressive repetition, flex the muscle harder and create your own resistance, using an imaginary weight. This is one of the best ways to learn exercise perfection.

3. Never get stuck in an exercise rut or allow yourself to get bored with a workout. Your body thrives on variety. You should rotate routines regularly and try to use a wide variety of different angles, exercises, and equipment to stimulate the muscles and other body systems. I have provided several different routines that can help you to always keep things interesting for the body and for the mind.

4. Never throw the weights around during an exercise. There should be nothing at all ballistic about any exercise described in this book. If you train at a gym and see others working out with sloppy form, doing fast, bouncing reps, don't copy

them. They're doing it wrong. Think of your exercises as moving in slow motion. Keep control of the weight at all times, throughout every rep. Let others copy your style, after they see the results that you're getting from exercise perfection and controlled execution.

5. Never use more weight than you can handle with good form on any exercise. Using body momentum is only a road to injury. And injury will sidetrack your efforts. Don't arch your back to get that last Bench Press rep; don't squirm around to crank out that last Biceps Curl. If you can't get the reps with good form, lower the weight on the next set.

6. "Hang your ego at the gym door." This is a motto that I've used for the past 20 years. You aren't in the gym to compete against anyone. You are there to get your own body into shape. Use your training as a martial-arts master would use his: as a blend of physical effort combined with an almost meditative concentration and focus. Give every rep, set, and workout your full attention. When you use your mind along with your body, you create a synergistic impact that multiplies gains.

7. Use your observation skills to learn when your body has had enough. Know the difference between the bad pain of a potential injury and the good pain of muscle burn caused by intense contractions.

8. Keep your workouts moving. Don't rest too long between sets. In fact, if you train alone, rest only 30 seconds to one minute between sets—just enough time to begin to catch your breath. If you train with a partner, rest only long enough for the partner to do a set. Always keep it moving. Slow, controlled reps, but fast and brief workouts. That's the key to results.

9. Watch out for the most vulnerable areas of the body, like your lower back, elbows, and knees. Know what is injured and where you are vulnerable. If an exercise hurts and you've done everything possible to perfect the form, try something different. Unless you're working with an injury, if you use the techniques described here and really focus, you should remain injury-free. Remember, though, that as your body ages it becomes more vulnerable to aches and pains. Take this into account when deciding on your training and recovery times.

10. Give your muscles adequate rest between intense workouts. In general, a muscle that's trained to positive failure and with strong intensity takes between two and three days to recuperate. Body parts shouldn't be worked every day with

weight-training exercises. Recovery from an isometric routine will be faster, but you should still pay attention to any muscle soreness and take steps to recover.

STRENGTHEN YOUR HEART AND LUNGS

1. Warm up thoroughly for your cardio workouts. In many of the routines in this book, stretching will be used as a means of getting the blood flowing. No matter what, you should begin slowly and let your body come up to speed. This may mean using a lighter tension setting or a slower speed, but do not just launch in without allowing the system to become accustomed to the exercise for at least two or three minutes. Avoid that very male tendency to want to just get right at it. Begin slowly and find your stride.

2. Monitor your heart rate every few minutes. It's easy to allow the body to pick up the pace to too intense a level, or to move without proper intensity and let the heart rate slip. Know your target range before you start out, and stay there once your body is warmed up.

3. Break out of the mindset that views any type of exercise as a competition or an attempt to break a world record. The purpose of your cardio is very specific and goal-oriented. This exercise is purely for your own benefit. Keep your heart rate inside the target range.

4. If you become light-headed or dizzy, stop the exercise. Don't push through. Get off the machine and sit down. Drink some water and catch your breath. You can begin to do some stretching exercises when you start to recover. Use common sense as to whether or not you should continue your cardio exercise. If you stand up and feel dizzy again, stop. Pay attention to the signals that your body sends you.

5. Concentrate on the exercise that you're doing. Pay attention to the form that you use. Don't bounce or jar your joints. Imagine that you're gliding in a smooth and steady way. Use good posture. When you power-walk, stand up straight and push off with your legs and glutes; keep your head up. Using good exercise posture will trigger your mind in a postitive way.

6. Find a way to use your mind as you exercise. There are many options. The most obvious is to listen to music to pass the time. The other is to read (if you're on a machine). I feel that these should be second and third choices. Yes, cardio can seem boring, and the time can pass slowly, if you don't direct it. I like to develop

a few positive affirmations to repeat as I do my cardio. The more you tie the various aspects of your body together (body and mind, for example), the more tuned-in to your efforts you become. Yes, it may be simple to try and distract yourself with tapes or magazines, but it's also a way of subtly saying that the activity doesn't deserve your full attention. Remember, attention is key to success. Read or listen to music if it means the difference between doing cardio and not doing it, but also give active meditation, affirmations, and visualization—give your imagination—a chance.

7. Don't push yourself for too long. At 60 percent (the low end of your heart-rate range), an hour should be the maximum length of your cardio workout (assuming that you're in reasonable condition). At 70 percent, 40 minutes is the upper limit. You want your body to be able to recover in a timely manner from what you're doing.

8. If you are an absolute beginner who's been inactive for a long time, begin very slowly. Take a walk around the block. Next time, walk around two blocks. Before you know it—if you follow the advice in this book—you'll be power-walking four or five miles and longing for more. Build your fitness life one step at a time, and remember that results are cumulative.

BUILD FLEXIBILITY

1. Always strive to make the muscles feel long. Use both your physical body and your imagination while you're executing a stretch. As you reach out, for example, see the muscles—and the places where you feel resistance and tightness—elongate and lengthen. By blending physical effort with directed imagination, you can make the stretch much more effective.

2. Never bounce or jerk your body into any stretched position. If you find that you are doing this, stop. Focus your full attention on making the movement slow and steady. Go into the stretch over the course of several seconds. Breathe deeply and relax. Doing this will enable your body to slow down and relax further, and that will make it more flexible.

3. Make the time. Plan any workout so that you integrate the time to build your body's flexibility. You should set aside a minimum of five to ten minutes for stretching. And, since many of the *Prime* routines will include Power Stretches, it's important that you don't skip them. The routines are carefully designed for maximum benefit.

4. Record your stretching in your journal. Write down how you felt about what you were doing—including if you thought it was a waste of time (which it clearly is not). Write about how your body felt, including where your tight spots were and which area was the most difficult. Recording this information may seem to be a pain, but you'll be surprised by how happy you'll be when you're able to review your progress and analyze what worked and what didn't. Always keep a written record.

5. Never push beyond the point of maximum tension in a stretch. Be patient with your body. Your flexibility will increase with time and effort. You don't need to be as flexible as a yoga master today. Elongate your muscles to the point of tension, breathe, and go a bit farther if you can.

6. Hold your stretches and breathe in a relaxed way. Let your mind become calm and focused. Keep the stretch at a maximum extension for the amount of time recommended. If this feels too long, you may be pushing the stretch too hard. Relax. It isn't a competition. Don't be one of those men who hold their stretches for two or three seconds and thinks he's done all he can do. Find the calmness inside to make your body still.

7. If you have an area that is injured, go very slowly at first. Don't push hard, and yet don't avoid the area. This is one of those paradoxical balancing points about all fitness. You want to push, but also simultaneously ease up. This is where learning how your unique body works comes in handy, and it's especially true when it comes to unique quirks, such as injuries or particularly tight areas. If you can move only an inch, do that. And then when you return again, you'll be able to do a bit more.

8. Be very careful with the vulnerable parts of your body. Areas such as the lower back, the area where the chest and shoulders tie together, the knees and elbows—these need to be shown respect for their current condition. You can only go forward from where you are now. If you've allowed yourself to become inflexible, you must move into a new era with a quiet respect for where you are in life right this minute.

9. Never take your flexibility for granted. It must be reinforced with regular, consistent practice. If you are limber now, look at an investment in your flexibility as an asset in which you must constantly reinvest. The body does not stay static. What is in shape today will dwindle tomorrow if you neglect it. On the other hand, what has dwindled can be built back up today with knowledge and action.

10. As you stretch, use the visualization, relaxation, and affirmation techniques discussed in MOTIVATED MIND to maximize your efforts. You can multiply your fitness and wellness results by working at several different levels. By relaxing your mind, and by using it to reinforce your positive imagery, you create a positive, upward loop that will lead to a greater quality of life.

CREATE ROUTINES

The best inspiration is not to outdo others, but to outdo ourselves.
—ANONYMOUS

BASIC FLEXIBILITY SEQUENCE #1

PURPOSE
can be used to warm up before any resistance or cardio workout

EXPERIENCE LEVEL
all levels

INTENSITY
relaxed

PERFORMANCE SPEED
move slowly into all stretches; hold each one for at least 20 counts

REPETITIONS
1 stretch per side, per movement

SETS
beginners 1 time through; more advanced as needed

REST TIME
move from one stretch to the next without rest

RECOVERY TIME
can be done every day, assuming no existing injuries

The Workout

1. Neck Roll (front, back, and sides)

2. Chest/Biceps Stretch (for each side)

3. Back Stretch (for each side)

4. Shoulder/Triceps Towel Stretch (for each side)

5. Head-to-Knee Stretch (for each side)

6. Forward Bend

BASIC FLEXIBILITY SEQUENCE #2

PURPOSE
Develops a more advanced level of flexibility, agility, balance, and a bit of muscle strength. Also can be an excellent warmup routine before a cardio or natural body builder routine.

EXPERIENCE LEVEL
beginners with recent athletic experience (otherwise, begin with 1 week of Sequence #1 before moving to this one), intermediate and advanced

INTENSITY
can be done in a very relaxed style for a calming effect or in a more vigorous style to stimulate the system. The vigorous style is a great wake-up.

PERFORMANCE SPEED
movements should be slow, steady, and fully controlled

REPETITIONS
1 stretch per movement

SETS
1 time through the sequence for beginners (or when used as a warmup); up to 3 times through for the more advanced, depending on use. As a warmup for other exercises, 1 time through.

REST TIME
move without rest from one movement to the next all the way through

depends upon intensity. Generally can be done every day; however, if done in an intense style for more than 2 sets, it may require a full rest day before repeating.

The Workout

1. Warm up: For each side, do the Chest/Biceps Stretch, then the Towel Triceps/Shoulder Stretch, then Head-to-Knee Stretch, then Cross Leg Twist.

2. Stand with the feet in a wide stance. Do Neck Rolls, front, back and sides.

3. With the eyes straight ahead, go slowly into a Wide Leg Stretch.

4. Roll the spine back to the upright position.

5. Put the arms out to the sides and twist the trunk in one direction into Warrior II.

6. Twist the trunk in the opposite direction and repeat.

7. Twist back in the opposite direction into Warrior I.

8. Twist the trunk in the opposite direction and repeat.

9. Turn back to the front, arms extended to the sides.

10. Roll the spine into Wide Leg Stretch and roll back up.

11. Reach one hand to the opposite ankle and bend into Back Stretch.

12. Release and roll up; repeat Back Stretch in opposite direction.

13. When upright, bring the feet together, squat and lie face-down on the floor.

14. Slowly do Locust.

15. Come up onto the knees and slowly move into Camel.

BASIC FLEXIBILITY AND ISOMETRICS SEQUENCE #1

PURPOSE

to develop muscle tone and basic flexibility without weights; this is also an excellent workout to do when traveling.

EXPERIENCE LEVEL

beginner to advanced

INTENSITY

can be adjusted from moderate to very intense

PERFORMANCE SPEED

4 counts to contraction; 4 counts during flex; 4 counts to stretch

REPETITIONS

15 to 20 per exercise; 1 each on the stretches (for each side, as applicable)

SETS

for beginners, 1 to 2 sets; advanced 2 to 4 sets

REST TIME

only long enough to slightly catch your breath between exercises

RECOVERY TIME

1 to 2 days; the routine can be done by most men every other day

The Workout

WARMUP

Basic Flexibility and Isometrics Sequence #1

THEN DO IN SEQUENCE

Ballet Squat Isometric

Towel Leg Press/Row Isometric

Towel Pull-Down/Press Isometric

Towel Side Raise Isometric

Push-Up

Chest Press Isometric

Bench Dip

Towel Biceps/Triceps

Abdominal Crunch

Lying Leg Raise

COOLDOWN
Basic Flexibility Sequence #1

FLEXIBILITY AND ISOMETRICS SEQUENCE #2

PURPOSE

to warm up muscles and as a quick energy burst. This is an excellent pre-cardio warmup to get the heart rate elevated and muscles moving.

EXPERIENCE LEVEL

all levels

INTENSITY

should be done with a very focused and sure intensity, flexing muscles very hard throughout

PERFORMANCE SPEED

move as if in slow motion. 3 to 4 counts when moving; hold all muscle contractions for 10 to 20 counts

REPETITIONS

one of each movement through the full sequence is one rep. Do 8 to 10 reps per set. The entire sequence should flow together as one movement.

SETS

1 to 4, depending on use and level. Beginners should do 1 to 2. More advanced can do up to 4; less if it is a warmup for another resistance work-out.

REST TIME

between sets of sequence reps, enough time to barely catch breath; probably 20 to 30 seconds

RECOVERY TIME

can be used daily

The Workout

1. Assume the start position of the Ballet Squat Isometric.

2. Put the arms out to the sides, parallel to the ground.

3. Carefully bend the knees into the Ballet Squat Isometric.

4. Hold for a count of 10.

5. Slowly raise the arms straight overhead into a Pull-Down/Press. Isometric.

6. Using imaginary resistance, slowly pull the arms down.

7. Again using imaginary resistance, slowly press the arms back up.

8. Press the hands together and bring them straight down in front of the chest.

9. Push the hands together to begin Chest Press Isometric.

10. Slowly bring the hands back toward the chest, keeping constant tension.

11. Pushing against imaginary resistance, press the hands back out.

12. Bring the extended arms back out to the sides and stand up to the start position.

POWER FLEX

POWER FLEX WORKOUT 1

PURPOSE

develops a balanced blend of strength, flexibility, stamina, and focus. Will develop a sleeker body look (assuming proper nutrition) that isn't bulky.

EXPERIENCE LEVEL

suitable for all levels, so long as exercise-perfection techniques are used

INTENSITY

should be done with vigor

PERFORMANCE SPEED

resistance and isometric Exercises should be performed with 4 counts to contraction, 3 counts in the contraction position, and 4 counts back to stretch—in other words, very slowly. All stretches should be held for a minimum of 20 counts (each side, if applicable).

REPETITIONS

resistance and isometrics—10 to 20 reps (until positive failure); stretches—1 hold on each side per sequence

SETS

beginners, 1 time through; more advanced can do up to 4 times through the sequence, depending on conditioning

REST TIME

very little or no rest between exercises (unless uncomfortably out of breath) and less than 30 seconds between sets of the sequence; should be in continuous, controlled movement

RECOVERY TIME

can be done every other day, up to 3 times per week. Absolute beginners may need 2 days rest between workouts, depending on level of initial conditioning.

The Workout

Chest/Biceps Stretch

Push-Up

Chest Press Isometric

Warrior I

Two-Arm Dumbbell Row

Back Stretch

Towel Pull-Down/Press Isometric

Warrior II

Squat with Dumbbells

Ballet Squat Isometric

Wide Leg Stretch

Abdominal Crunch

Locust

POWER FLEX WORKOUT #2

PURPOSE
same as Workout #1

EXPERIENCE LEVEL
not for beginners; intermediate and advanced only

INTENSITY
high; should be done in a vigorous manner

PERFORMANCE SPEED
same as Workout #1

REPETITIONS
same as Workout #1

SETS
Workout #1 was done as a sequence; this one is done in a more traditional style—one exercise at a time.

REST TIME
a maximum of 15 seconds between sets, or the minimum time needed to move to the next exercise if done in a gym

RECOVERY TIME
usually one to two days

The Workout

Chest/Biceps Stretch

Incline Dumbbell Press

Chest Press Isometric

Camel

Wide-Grip Front Pull-Down

Back Stretch

Locust

Towel Shoulder/Triceps Stretch

Dumbbell Side Raise

Towel Side Raise Isometric

Biceps/Triceps Towel Stretch

Bench Dip

Dumbbell Curl

Chest/Biceps Stretch

Squat

Head-to-Knee Stretch

Leg Curl

Forward Bend

Ballet Squat Isometric

Lying Leg Raise

Additional Power Flex Tips

■ Use light weights for the resistance exercises and really squeeze the muscles as hard as you can on every rep. I recommend that most men use between 15- and 20-pound dumbbells. Create the stimulation and intensity through controlling the movement, not through the amount of weight used.

■ Move quickly between exercises, but within the exercises themselves, move as if in slow motion. Remember: slow, controlled reps. That's the only way to get the most out of this routine. Rushing through fast, sloppy reps and doing half-hearted stretches will simply waste your time and effort.

■ When you can, use a mirror to make sure you're doing the exercises correctly. Work on the more difficult, yoga-like stretches beforehand—sort of like a rehearsal—and then integrate them into your workout.

■ The time to do cardio exercise is immediately after your Power Flex workout, while your heart rate is elevated—if you have the energy and time. If you don't, do a cardio workout on the day between your Power Flex workouts. Warm up with one of the Basic Flexibility Sequences. In either case, do a minimum of 15 minutes of cardio in the 60-percent heart-rate range.

■ On the day between these Power Flex workouts, do one of the Basic Flexibility Sequences to stay limber, even if you choose not to do an off-day cardio work-out.

MUSCLE BLAST

MUSCLE BLAST #1 THROUGH #3

PURPOSE
a brief yet intense combination of compound resistance exercises, isometrics, and stretches, used to stimulate muscular response

EXPERIENCE LEVEL
beginner to advanced

INTENSITY

PERFORMANCE SPEED

resistance and isometric exercises are done with 4 counts to contraction, 2 counts to flex, and 4 counts to return to stretch. Stretches are held for a minimum of 20 counts (each side, as appropriate).

REPETITIONS

resistance exercise weights are adjusted to allow for 12 to 15 reps on the first set (as a warmup) and 8 to 10 reps on any additional sets. Stretches should be repeated twice for the above performance speed (for each side, as appropriate).

SETS

beginners, do 1 warmup set and 1 additional set. Advanced, do 1 warmup set and 2 to 3 additional sets. The exercises (resistance, isometric, and stretch) are performed in a tri-set (see Build Muscle).

REST TIME

no rest inside the tri-set. Minimal rest between full sets and exercises.

RECOVERY TIME

generally, 2 days of rest between workouts are needed if maximum intensity is used.

MUSCLE BLAST #1
The Workout

WARMUP
Basic Flexibility Sequence #1

AS A TRI-SET
Incline Barbell Press

Chest Press Isometric

Chest/Biceps Stretch

AS A TRI-SET
Leg Press

Ballet Squat Isometric

Camel

AS A TRI-SET
Wide-Grip Front Pull-Down

Towel Pull-Down/Press Isometric

Back Stretch

AS A TRI-SET
Abdominal Crunch

Lying Leg Raise

Locust

FOLLOWED BY
20 to 30 minutes of cardio at 60 percent

COOLDOWN
Basic Flexibility Sequence #1

MUSCLE BLAST #2
The Workout

WARMUP
Basic Flexibility Sequence #1

AS A TRI-SET
Flat Barbell Bench Press

Chest Press Isometric

Chest/Biceps Stretch

AS A TRI-SET
Back Squat

Towel Leg Press/Row Isometric

Head-to-Knee Stretch

AS A TRI-SET
Low Pulley Row

Towel Curl/Push-Down

Back Stretch

AS A TRI-SET
Abdominal Crunch

Warrior I

Warrior II

FOLLOWED BY
20 to 30 minutes of cardio at 60 percent

COOL-DOWN
Basic Flexibility Sequence #1

MUSCLE BLAST #3
The Workout

WARMUP
Basic Flexibility Sequence #1

AS A TRI-SET
Incline Dumbbell Press

Push-Up

Chest/Biceps Stretch

AS A TRI-SET
Two-Dumbbell Row

Towel Pull-Down/Press Isometric

Back Stretch

AS A TRI-SET
Back Squat

Ballet Squat Isometric

Wide Leg Stretch

AS A TRI-SET
Lying Leg Raise

Towel Curl/Push-down

Bridge

FOLLOWED BY
20 to 30 minutes of cardio at 60 percent

COOL-DOWN
Basic Flexibility Sequence #1

Additional Muscle Blast Tips

1. You must be getting plenty of rest for this routine to work well. Be sure your sleep is consistent and of good quality.

2. For this to really work, your nutrition should follow the plan coming up in Sound Nutrition.

3. Be sure to use the warmup sets carefully and fully. You must not jump straight into intense weight training without a proper warmup. The injuries that could result would sideline your efforts.

4. Rotate the three different workouts. Your body will thrive on variety. So will your mind. If you're bored with a workout, the results will be diminished.

5. Set your equipment up so that you can go from one exercise of the tri-set to the next with almost no rest.

NATURAL BODY BUILDER

NATURAL BODY BUILDER #1, OPTIONS A AND B

PURPOSE

a more traditional approach to developing muscle mass and size in a balanced way

EXPERIENCE LEVEL

beginning and intermediate

INTENSITY

moderate to high

PERFORMANCE SPEED

3 to 4 counts to contraction; hold flex for 1 to 2 counts; 3 to 4 counts to stretch

REPETITIONS

15 to 20 at a lower weight for the first set as a warmup. Then 10 to 15 on all other sets

SETS

2 sets per exercise for beginners; 3 sets per exercise for intermediates

REST TIME

45 seconds between sets; if training with a partner, the length of time it takes for the partner to do a set.

RECOVERY TIME

1 to 2 days; can be done 2 to 3 times per week depending on recovery time

Option A—The Workout

WARMUP

Basic Flexibility Sequence #1

RESISTANCE EXERCISES

Incline Barbell Press

Dumbbell Shoulder Press

Barbell Row

Bench Dip

Barbell Curl

Barbell Wrist Curl

Good Morning

Back Squat

Lying Leg Curl

Standing Calf Raise

Abdominal Crunch

THEN DO
15 to 20 minutes of cardio at 60–70 percent

COOL-DOWN
Basic Flexibility Sequence #1

Option B—The Workout

WARMUP
Basic Flexibility Sequence #1

RESISTANCE EXERCISES
Flat Barbell Bench Press

Wide-Grip Front Pull-Down

Behind-the-Neck Barbell Press

Dumbbell Curl

Triceps Push-Down

Leg Press

Lying Leg Curl

Hyperextension

Standing Calf Raise

Lying Leg Raise

THEN DO
15 to 20 minutes of cardio at 60 to 70 percent

NATURAL BODY BUILDER #2, OPTIONS A AND B

PURPOSE

an advanced yet basic and traditional approach to developing muscle mass and size

EXPERIENCE LEVEL

intermediate and advanced

INTENSITY

very high; all but warmup sets taken to positive failure

PERFORMANCE SPEED

3 to 4 counts to contraction; hold flex for 1 to 2 counts; 3 to 4 counts to stretch

REPETITIONS

15 to 20 at a lower weight for the first set as a warmup. Then 10 to 15 for the second set and 6 to 8 repetitions for the third set. Weight should be adjusted accordingly. Calf and abdominal exercises should be done in 15 to 20-rep sets for all 3 sets.

SETS

3 sets per exercise

REST TIME

45 seconds between sets, or the length of time it takes for a partner to do a set

RECOVERY TIME

2 to 3 days; workouts should be done with a rest day between Day One and Day Two routines in order to maximize gains

Option A: Day One

WARMUP

Basic Flexibility Sequence #1

RESISTANCE EXERCISES: CHEST

Incline Barbell Press

Flat Fly

Push-Up

RESISTANCE EXERCISES: SHOULDERS

Dumbbell Side Raise

Behind-the-Neck Barbell Press

RESISTANCE EXERCISES: TRICEPS

Triceps Push-Down

Bench Dip

RESISTANCE EXERCISE: CALVES

Standing Calf Raise

RESISTANCE EXERCISE: ABS

Abdominal Crunch

THEN DO

15 to 20 minutes of cardio at 70 percent

COOLDOWN

Basic Flexibility Sequence #1

Day Two

WARMUP

Basic Flexibility Sequence #1

RESISTANCE EXERCISES: BACK

Wide-Grip Front Pull-Down

Two-Dumbbell Row

Good Morning

RESISTANCE EXERCISES: BICEPS
Seated Two-Dumbbell Curl

Barbell Curl

RESISTANCE EXERCISE: FOREARMS
Barbell Wrist Curl

RESISTANCE EXERCISE: FRONT THIGHS
Leg Extension

Barbell Squat

RESISTANCE EXERCISE: HAMSTRINGS
Lying Leg Curl

THEN DO
15 to 20 minutes of cardio at 60 percent

COOLDOWN
Basic Flexibility Sequence #1

Option B: Day One

WARMUP
Basic Flexibility Sequence #1

RESISTANCE EXERCISES: CHEST
Incline Dumbbell Press

Incline Fly

Dip

RESISTANCE EXERCISES: SHOULDERS
Dumbbell Press

Seated Bent-Over Dumbbell Side Raise

RESISTANCE EXERCISES: TRICEPS
Lying Dumbbell Extension

Close-Grip Bench Press

RESISTANCE EXERCISE: CALVES

Seated Calf Raise

RESISTANCE EXERCISE: ABS

Lying Leg Raise

THEN DO

15 to 20 minutes of cardio at 70 percent

COOLDOWN

Basic Flexibility Sequence #1

Option B: Day Two

WARMUP

Basic Flexibility Sequence #1

RESISTANCE EXERCISE: BACK

Wide-Grip Behind-the-Neck Pull-Down

RESISTANCE EXERCISES: BICEPS

Alternating Two-Dumbbell Curl

Two-Arm Machine (or Pulley) Curl

RESISTANCE EXERCISE: FOREARMS

Two-Dumbbell Wrist Curl

RESISTANCE EXERCISES: FRONT THIGHS

Leg Extension

Leg Press

RESISTANCE EXERCISE: HAMSTRINGS

Lying Leg Curl

THEN DO

15 to 20 minutes of cardio at 60 percent

COOLDOWN

Basic Flexibility Sequence #1

Additional Natural Body Builder Tips

1. Alternate Options A and B for each workout day. Take at least one full day of rest between the workouts. It you're not recovering fully with one day off, take two until the body catches up. Pay close attention to your body's signals, such as extreme soreness and fatigue.

2. On the off-days I recommend doing one of the Basic Flexibility Sequences in addition to doing some guided relaxation and visualization exercises.

3. Don't skip the flexibility sequences or the cardio workouts on training days. If you do, you won't achieve the fullest benefits from the program. With this program, you should not do cardio on days off.

4. Be sure to observe all of the rules of exercise performance. These programs were designed to be unique in repetition style. The old-fashioned method of slinging weights isn't acceptable. Go slow and squeeze. Feel everything.

5. Be sure to utilize the affirmation and visualization exercises discussed in MOTI-VATED MIND. These can play an important role in making the most of the workouts.

MAKE SMART ADJUSTMENTS

As you work to create new fitness habits, you'll learn something new about your body each day—if you pay attention.

Using your attention to how your body responds to exercise can help you to be sure the routines you are using are taking you toward your goals. Use your journal as a guide to how well your exercise has been going. If you've been diligent in recording your daily routines, you'll have a wealth of highly personalized knowledge to draw from.

Ask yourself these key questions:

Are there any areas that need more attention?

Am I on or off track in my efforts?

Can I be more diligent in my workouts?

Have I been observing the rules of exercise perfection?

Am I keeping myself injury-free?

Am I skipping over areas of the fitness programs?

Am I recovering effectively from the training?

Now go to your journal and, when you have a few minutes to focus, look at the goals that you've set for your body. Consider whether or not they need to be updated according to your latest understanding of how you react to exercise.

And above all else, be flexible. Make adjustments. Go back and reread the sections in this book that cover areas where your progress may be lacking. The most important things to consider—aside from attention and flexibility—are that this is an ongoing process, and that your efforts on behalf of your own fitness and wellness never go to waste.

PRIME

PART FOUR

SOUND NUTRITION

More die in the United States of too much food than of too little.

—JOHN KENNETH GALBRAITH

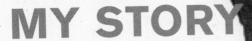

MY STORY

I began to train seriously in my late teens. I worked out with weights, but still consumed vast quantities of a typical teenager's diet— burgers, pizzas, milkshakes, and so on— added to the everyday country-style food I was raised eating: fried chicken, buttered and overcooked vegetables, pork chops, et cetera. This was all considered perfectly normal. It was how everyone around me ate, young and old.

My young metabolism simply burned it all up, and I stayed relatively lean while gaining muscle from my training. It wasn't until I began to consider competing as a bodybuilder that I educated myself about the importance of good nutrition. I quickly learned that, if I wanted to succeed at the sport I'd chosen, I was going to need to cut out the junk food and the high-fat "deep-fried everything" foods of my youth.

I became ultra-disciplined with my eating and stayed that way all through my competitive years. I didn't have a choice. Given that one of the criteria for success in my sport was ultra-low body-fat, I needed to change my eating habits or I'd fail. The disciplined eating became second nature. It wasn't easy; most of the time I wished that it could be different—that I could return to the comfortable foods of my youth—but reality was what it was and I sustained the habit.

When I retired from competition, I could once again eat anything that I wanted. While I didn't return to eating fried catfish sandwiches, barbecued pork, and the like for lunch every day, I did loosen my diet considerably. This wasn't a good move on my part. I had a metabolism that kept me kind of lean, but other factors suffered. Besides experiencing a rise in cholesterol and blood pressure (which are both directly linked to poor dietary habits), I also began to feel as if I had a hangover the day after I ate heavy, fatty foods. My body was reacting to something that wasn't good for it, just as it would respond to too much liquor.

When I set about rediscovering my fitness goals as a grown man, seeking not competitive goals but great health, I began to retool my diet. I returned to the discoveries that I'd made early on in my training days, but geared them to my current life and goals. I took into account the foods that were going to keep me growing healthier as I aged. I ate things that I would never have imagined eating when I was a young man, but I had to. I didn't want to die early because of my own bad eating habits, nor did I want to suffer from miserable health along the way just so I could eat junk food. The sacrifice (and it was only a sacrifice at the very beginning) was well worth it. I feel amazing now, and I look at least 10 years younger than I did when I was eating whatever came my way. I'll trade in corn fritters and french fries for this feeling any day of the week.

EAT YOUR WAY TO HEALTH

If inactivity is the direct road to the decline of physical strength, then inattention to diet is the fast track to a host of health problems that can be rather easily counteracted. The problem lies in our culture. The way we approach food in general is oriented toward convenience and pleasure rather than nourishment and health.

I'm not the first person to point out that our modern diet, with its emphasis on massive portions and heavy fat, is killing us—or at the very least making our lives miserable. Think about it: How can a man live on a diet of bacon-double-cheeseburgers and glazed doughnuts and then wonder why, once he's reached middle age, he's overweight and having the beginnings of health problems ranging from diabetes to heart disease to cancer? If I sound a bit hard-edged about this, it's only because I feel so strongly that—along with smoking—poor diet is a fundamental way for a man to all but guarantee that the second half of his life will be more difficult, and certainly more unhealthy, than it needs to be.

The good news in all of this, however, is that the counteraction to these health and weight concerns are within a man's control—if he's willing to take an honest look at his current habits and make some serious changes. And I have some more good news: Even though many men think that nutrition is complicated, it's actually very simple. I didn't say that eating right was easy—especially if you're overcoming entrenched bad habits. I said that it was simple. In fact, of the three Key Elements in the *Prime* program, SOUND NUTRITION is by far the simplest. It consists of only three basic ideas, which are:

Don't Diet, Eat Clean

Eat These 70 Clean Foods

Supplement Intelligently

IDENTIFY
THE NEED

Within each experience of pain or negativity is the opportunity to challenge the perception that lies behind it.

—GARY ZUKAV

Here are a few examples of challenges and hurdles that may stand between a 40+ man and his integration of SOUND NUTRITION.

Please remember that, while many of these challenges may initially sound sort of "negative," we must first name something to claim it. Identify the Need first, then seek an informed solution. My goal is to get you to start thinking about your own situation in a deeper way.

See if you can identify some of your own needs below:

- A man finds himself constantly struggling to keep his weight under control.

- He believes that he can solve his weight problem fast by using some gimmicky but unbalanced short-term diet he hears or reads about.

- Each time he uses a gimmick diet, he finds himself rebounding to a condition even more out-of-shape than before.

- He finds that, with age, this yo-yo approach—even with the strictest of gimmick diets—stops working at all.

- His doctor has told him that he needs to lose weight, but he doesn't know how.

- He hears a lot of contradictory information about what he should eat and it goes in one ear and out the other.

- He finds himself simply grabbing whatever is fast and easy.

- He reacts to stress with a constant junk-food diet.

- He hasn't got a clue about which foods are actually good for him.

- He eats massive portions at every meal.

- He skips breakfast, and then out of sheer starvation he grabs the first thing he can find and stuffs himself on it.

- He belongs to the Clean Plate Club.

- He can't keep himself from stuffing his face with junk in the evening.

- He can't remember the last time he drank a glass of plain water.

- He drinks mainly coffee and soda.

- He never takes vitamins, even though he knows that his dietary habits stink.

- He flips through a fitness magazine and believes what the ads for many of those supplements say—that there's a miracle pill or potion out there.

- He has wasted tons of money in the past on supplements that did nothing.

- He doesn't really know what he should take and what he should avoid.

ESTABLISH YOUR PERSPECTIVE

It's time once again to play 20 Questions. As in MOTIVATED MIND and FIT BODY, I strongly encourage you to write your answers and further observations in your journal. Do this exercise when you have plenty of time to focus. Breathe yourself into a nice, relaxed place, and really give yourself the chance to honestly explore where you are with these issues related to your approach to SOUND NUTRITION.

Allow me to remind you that this is a rather unique approach to this information, and that the answers to these questions should be used to deepen your self-understanding, not as a test in which you can get something right or wrong.

The answers that you come up with should give you insight into where you are and how you feel. They are essentially meditation points, more than anything truly rigid and concrete.

After you've given the following 20 questions due consideration, I encourage you to bring that enlightened perspective to the next sections—which will then hopefully help your knowledge grow and evolve.

QUESTION 1: Do you feel as if you understand the basics of nutrition?

QUESTION 2: What do you usually do if you're feeling overweight or flabby?

QUESTION 3: Pertaining to your answer to Question 2: In your head, do you consider this a quick fix?

QUESTION 4: Does your body still respond in the same ways to a diet such as this as it would have when you were younger?

QUESTION 5: Do you tend to revert to old habits after ending a diet?

QUESTION 6: What does your typical day's menu look like?

QUESTION 7: Is this way of eating contributing to or taking away from your health and fitness?

QUESTION 8: Do you feel "hooked" on any particular foods (especially junk foods)?

QUESTION 9: What would it feel like to go without those foods?

QUESTION 10: How did your family eat when you were growing up?

QUESTION 11: Have you continued those habits as an adult?

QUESTION 12: What is the time of day when you're most vulnerable to eating foods that aren't good for you?

QUESTION 13: Do you tend to eat more when you're already completely full?

QUESTION 14: Do you spread your meals consistently throughout the day?

QUESTION 15: Do you ever experience a dizzy, light-headed feeling between meals?

QUESTION 16: How many glasses of plain water do you drink each day on a consistent basis?

QUESTION 17: What has your experience been with vitamins and minerals?

QUESTION 18: Have you ever invested in an expensive supplement program and been disappointed with the results?

QUESTION 19: When you go into a vitamin store, do you understand what all of those shelves of supplements are for?

QUESTION 20: Has your doctor ever told you that you need to change your way of eating?

GATHER THE FACTS

Give a man a fish and you feed him for a day.
Teach a man to fish and you feed him for a lifetime.
—CHINESE PROVERB

DON'T DIET

When it comes to nutrition, the majority of men fall into one of two categories. They either don't pay any attention to nutrition at all and eat whatever they feel like, which is usually junk food, or they bounce back and forth between eating that way (what's rapidly becoming something of a cultural norm) and some version of the latest gimmicky miracle diet. If you're 40+ and fall into either of these two categories, you are probably noticing that both have significant price tags.

With most men, the first version (the old high-fat, high-sugar, drive-thru diet) really begins to take its toll when the late 30s roll around; by 40 it almost feels too late. The belly grows bigger with each passing year; the body grows more sluggish. And those cholesterol and blood-pressure numbers are going up way too fast.

The man with the bouncer's approach is getting much the same result—and it may be worse—because whenever he goes on another crash miracle diet (his aunt swore that a low-carbohydrate bacon-and-butter diet was a sure thing!), he can't keep the weight off; in fact, with each passing year, the fat seems to get more and more stubborn—nearly impossible to drop. Then, after that quick fix ends, the inevitable rebound leads to even more fat and even more frustration, in a seemingly endless no-win loop. Why even try, right?

Your metabolism—the way your body burns the food you eat—is slowing down. That's a simple fact of growing older. What you could get away with in your teens and twenties will hurt you today, if you don't make a change. And all those bacon-double-cheeseburgers are clogging up your arteries and generally fouling up the machinery of your body—and they're going to all but ensure that your health becomes miserable.

But "dieting," in the traditional, quick-fix ways that are so popular these days, isn't the way to change things. Why? Two simple reasons:

■ Most gimmick diets—the ones that promise fast weight loss—are so unbalanced and extreme in food composition and calorie levels that they are simply unsustainable. If you eat, for example, one of those extremely low-carbohydrate diets that are the leading fad right now, you will spend every minute with cravings that only a binge can satisfy. You can't keep it up, and you'll be counting the minutes until the diet is over and you can get back to "normal." Such a diet is designed only to be a quick fix and therefore misses the point—which is much more than simple, temporary weight loss—almost entirely.

■ Many of the other gimmicky diets are completely unconcerned with the health issues that are central to the 40+ man, such as cholesterol, blood pressure, and colon cancer. They simply strive to turn the unhealthy eating habits that a man already has into a method of weight loss. This is an approach that is bound for failure, if some of the major criteria are an improvement in health, quality longevity, and long-term weight control. Diets that encourage you to focus on eating unhealthy foods (like bacon and butter) miss the point completely and cannot be sustained healthfully for the long term.

The only sustainable, healthy "diet" that any 40+ man—who is seeking not to merely lose a few quick pounds, but also to control his weight and improve his overall health—should pursue is a lifestyle change. That means a complete overhaul of the way he views food in his life. It isn't really as hard as it may sound at first. You simply must come to terms with the fact that how you eat has a direct impact on your health, and then make a choice to take charge of this issue. You are going to have to face the fact that no unbalanced, short-term, gimmicky diet is going to come along that will enable you to keep your health at its peak. You've got to make a one-day-at-a-time investment and keep it up day after day. It's that simple.

It's always a balancing act. The key reason that most gimmick diets don't work is that they don't try to address real and sustainable change. They aim for the buzz of a quick fix, and never tell you how to make the shift that will carry you beyond the limited time period of deprivation. As I've said before in this book, if you want to create a massive shift in your habits—replacing something harmful with something healthy—you must determine two things:

- What you need to get away from, or avoid

- What you must go toward, or embrace

As you revamp your outlook toward healthy eating—away from a poor diet and toward what I call Clean Eating—you'll need a set of rules for what to move away from and what to move toward. I've used this method for years, and most especially when I began my own *Prime* program and looked for the healthiest and most balanced way to put my nutrition on track. I call them my Rules for Clean Eating, and each one will include aspects of what to move away from and what to move toward.

THE RULES OF CLEAN EATING

Part One: Things to Move Away From

- Never Eat Unconsciously: Any time you aren't paying attention to what you are eating, you lose. Think of a time when you sat in front of the TV with some food and then a while later looked down and couldn't believe that you ate it all. The fastest path toward unhealthy eating habits is shutting your mind off and stuffing your face.

- **Never Skip Meals:** Many men skip breakfast and then grab something from a vending machine or drive-thru because they're so hungry that they'd eat anything in sight. Skipping meals assures that your blood sugar will drop through the floor. This will send signals to your brain that it needs fuel—any fuel—and you'll grab the first thing you can find, which will likely be junk.

- **Stop Overfeeding:** We live in a culture of plenty, yet people are dying from the impact of all that plenty. The surest way to become overweight is to keep eating beyond the point of hunger. Food meets so many men's emotional needs, acting as a substitute, in many cases, for something deeper. Combine that with the whole "super-size-it" fast-food culture, add the notion (one that so many of us were raised with) that you must clean your plate at every meal and that it is rude not to take second or third helpings, and an environment for ill health and ballooning weight is created.

- **Don't Obsessively Count Calories:** The converse of the overfeeding syndrome is the obsessive focus on calorie counting that so many men get into when they try to diet. Yes, calories are important, but they're only a part of the larger picture. And a dieter's over-focus on complex calorie calculations all but guarantees that the diet will fail, simply because constantly measuring and weighing foods and looking up their caloric values will become a hassle.

- **Avoid the Bad Fat:** In the burger-and-pizza culture, the average man is essentially eating an artery-clogging diet. You should know what constitutes the bad form of fat that's responsible for so many health problems that are relevant to your life. The killers are saturated, trans- and partially hydrogenated fats, which raise LDL (bad) cholesterol levels through the roof. The list of foods that contain the bad fats is a long one. You must stay away from butter, lard, most junk food (pizza, burgers, fries, et cetera), all deep-fried foods, dairy products (excluding not-fat varieties), fatty beef, all poultry skin, pork, bacon, and lamb. This is by no means a full list—these fats also appear in many packaged snack foods as well.

- **Cut Out Refined Sugar and Flour:** Table sugar and white flour (including bread that's made with processed flour) are foods that contribute nothing except empty calories to a man's diet. Other than taste, they bring nothing to the table except rapid rises and falls in blood sugar. A diet high in refined, simple sugar can also lead to diabetes (especially when combined with a sedentary, high-fat lifestyle). You should also stay away from honey (which the body treats as a simple sugar) and most of what commercial bread manufacturers call "wheat bread," which is mainly refined white flour dyed brown.

- Cut the Salt: Most men eat enough salt to pickle a barrel of fish. Having once been a salt-a-holic, I know how tough a habit it is to kick. But salt desensitizes the taste buds until you can't taste anything else. Almost all foods contain some sodium; I'm saying put away the salt-shaker. High salt usage leads to high blood pressure, which can lead to strokes and other health issues. Salt also makes the body retain a great deal of excess fluid, which leads to a puffy, bloated body.

Part Two: Things to Move Toward

- Pay Attention While Eating: Your meals should get your complete attention. The environment where you eat should be relaxed, and you should stay aware of each bite of food that you put into your mouth. Chew your food one bite at a time. Pause between bites and taste the food that you're eating. Attention and consciousness are the pathways to change in all elements of the *Prime* program—and this one is no exception.

- Spread Meals Throughout the Day: Plan your meals in advance. Begin eating when you get up in the morning (or whenever you get out of bed). Your body has been through a long period of fasting while you slept. I know it sounds sort of motherly, but eating breakfast is amazingly important in keeping your eating plan on track. You should eat a meal every three to four hours without fail. You have to plan for this. The number of meals that you eat during the day will depend on your current metabolism. Is it slow, medium, or fast? In other words, do you tend to get heavy easily (slow), stay the same (medium), or burn everything off and stay thin (fast)? Here's how it breaks down:

  Slow to medium metabolism: Eat 4 to 5 meals through the day.

  Fast metabolism: Eat 5 to 6 meals through the day.

- Eat Light: When I tell you to eat between 4 and 6 meals per day, I'm not talking about gut-busters. You should be eating meals that are on the small side. The latest medical research shows that men who live longest and healthiest tend to be lighter eaters. It isn't good for your system to be loaded down. Your meals should be balanced between the different food categories on the upcoming list. And forget about the hassles of overly measured quantities. There's an easier way. Use these guidelines for your portions:

  Meat, Fish, or Tofu: One portion is roughly the size of a pack of playing cards.

  Egg Whites: One portion is six whites.

  Starchy Complex Carbohydrates (rice, oats, beans, potatoes, etc.): One portion is roughly equal to the size of a balled-up fist.

Vegetables: One portion is roughly the size of a double-cupped handful.

Berries: One portion is roughly the size of a balled-up fist.

Other Fruits: One portion is the size of one medium piece of that particular fruit.

- Eat Some Good Fat: You definitely should not eliminate all fats from your diet. That would be nearly impossible anyway, especially when you use my food list. Your body needs what are known as the "good" fats, just not in unlimited quantities. Don't take this as permission to soak everything in olive oil, for example. A diet high in monounsaturated fats and a small amount of polyunsaturated fats tends to lower LDL (bad) cholesterol and may in fact raise the levels of HDL (good) cholesterol. Omega-6 fats boost a man's hormone, sight, and brain function, and they assist in holding the aging process at bay. Following the food chart that's coming up will assure you of getting all of these that you need.

  Good Oils (olive, etc): One daily portion should be limited to 1 tablespoon.

- Eat Lean Protein at Every Meal: Protein is the building block of muscles and cells. You must have an adequate protein supply with every meal to fuel your muscles and prevent the breakdown that occurs with aging. Just as protein is vital to the growing boy, so too is it essential to the aging man. You need not go overboard on the amounts, but you should have one portion of one of the listed lean protein sources with every single meal.

- Eat Complex Carbohydrates: Your number-one concern in life is energy—to be able to live, be active, and recuperate from exercise. Your body is reliant on the breakdown of complex carbohydrates for the energy that it needs, especially when you're training. Your muscles burn glycogen, which is the metabolite of carbohydrates and the fuel for your brain and other vital bodily functions. This is why low-carbohydrate diets are bound to fail—as a long-term nutrition plan— and why they lead to such violent cravings. Your brain and your body need the fuel that carbohydrates provide. You also need to get those carbohydrates from complex sources (those that break down more slowly and evenly than simple sugars) for the fiber, vitamins, and minerals provided by whole grains, legumes, beans, vegetables, and fruits, to both prevent disease and promote health.

- Appreciate Natural Flavors: When you eat clean and avoid salt, it will seem like a sacrifice at first, but your taste buds will return to full capacity. You'll be able to find the real flavor of the food that you eat. By cooking without salt, you have more freedom to experiment with other herbs and spices, and to discover new ways of cooking your clean foods.

- Drink a Lot of Water: This is one of the simplest concepts in the entire book and yet one of the most essential for keeping aging at bay and staying healthy. You must drink a lot of water throughout the day, every day. Period. Diet drinks aren't a replacement; neither is coffee, nor beer. Your body is made up of water. Seventy-five percent of the surface of the planet that you live on is water. Water is life. In our modern, convenient world, many of us men have forgotten the simple life connection of plain old H_2O. If you drink it, your skin will look better, you'll be more efficient in your exercise, and all of the systems of your body will be healthier.

- Use a Structure: Every one of your meals should be composed of:
    One portion of lean protein
    One portion of a starchy complex carbohydrate
    One portion of vegetables, after noon
    One portion of fruit or berries, before noon

USE THESE 70 FOODS

The key to building health is simple. As much as it is within your power, go away from the bad stuff and toward the good. This rather simple section is about a fundamental secret to building amazing health. As a side effect of using it—and by following the rules outlined above—you will also get a fantastic body.

The fundamental secret is that, simply by regularly including certain whole foods in your meals, you can turn your health around; you can get in the best shape of your life.

I have culled from all my nutrition journals, from all my years of training and learning how nutrition works, and I've come up with a list that makes Clean Eating simple.

There is one simple rule to making this work:

- Within the guidelines of balanced meals and portions listed in the rules of the previous section, you are to eat nothing that isn't on one of the two lists that follow. Every single meal that you eat should be made up of these 70 foods. Create your entire grocery list from these charts.

These two lists provide every food that you need to get in shape and reclaim your health. The first list is of my Top 10 picks of the foods that no man who is concerned about his health should ever be without. These foods are as close to miracles as you'll ever find.

They supply nutrients and vitamins and minerals that will boost the health of any man who makes a habit of eating (or drinking) them.

Do you believe me when I tell you that it's this simple? It is. I'm living proof. This system is the one that I used to turn my own fitness life around. I include each and every one of these foods on a daily basis in my own diet.

THE TOP 10 FOODS THAT EVERY 40+ MAN SHOULD EAT

FOOD ITEM	WHY WE NEED IT
TOMATOES	More than any other food, tomatoes are loaded with the cancer-fighting agent lycopene (which gives tomatoes their bright red color), which is even more potent than disease-fighting beta-carotene.
GREEN VEGETABLES	A great source of energy, they reduce the risk of stroke, are a great source of protein, and are loaded with vitamins A, B-complex, C, D, E, and K.
YAMS	Loaded with cancer preventive beta-carotene (vitamin A); a good source of folate, which is essential in the fight against heart disease; and they're fat-free.
OATMEAL (OR OAT BRAN)	Much more than just comfort food, oatmeal can reduce blood-cholesterol levels, lower blood pressure, and generally reduce the long-term risk of heart disease. Top a bowl of oats with blueberries and a better breakfast is almost impossible to find.
GARLIC	Contains 40 organic compounds that can lower blood pressure, promote better immunity; is also a great antioxidant source.
RED GRAPES (OR 1–2 SERVINGS OF RED WINE)	An amazing source of powerful antioxidants offering protection from heart disease and cancer by preventing LDL (bad) cholesterol from being oxidized into artery-clogging plaque, they also help prevent the formation of internal blood clots.
BLUEBERRIES	Absolutely the best source of antioxidant properties (one cup can double the average daily intake of antioxidants); therefore they have tremendous implications for the prevention of free-radical–related diseases.
FISH (SALMON, MACKEREL)	These fatty fish are incredibly rich in omega-3 polyunsaturated fatty acids. At least one serving per week can lower the risk of dying from a heart attack by 44 percent.
GREEN TEA	An extremely good source of antioxidants, green tea is reputed to be helpful in fighting cancer, rheumatoid arthritis, high cholesterol levels, cardiovascular disease, infection, and impaired immune function. What else do you need to know?
WATER	It is as miraculous as it is abundant. Water is beneficial to healthy skin and appearance; assists the body in metabolizing stored fat; relieves fluid retention; assists in maintaining proper muscle tone; helps carry nutrients through the blood and transports oxygen to the blood; rids the body of waste and toxins; reduces sodium buildup; and suppresses appetite.

THE OTHER 60 FOODS IN THE CLEAN EATING PLAN

VEGETABLES	WHY WE NEED IT
ARTICHOKES	High in fiber, cancer-fighting properties
AVOCADO	Vitamin E, high in monounsaturated fat that is beneficial to the heart
BEETS	Antioxidant properties
BOK CHOY	Good source of calcium and vitamin C
BROCCOLI	Packed with cancer-fighting components, calcium, folic acid, and vitamin C
BRUSSELS SPROUTS	Packed with vitamin C
CABBAGE	Fiber, cancer-fighting properties
CARROTS	Packed with beta-carotene (vitamin A)
CAULIFLOWER	High in fiber and vitamin C
CELERY	Compounds known to lower cholesterol and blood pressure
CORN	Contains the antioxidant selenium, which protects cells
GREEN BEANS	Loaded with antioxidants
GREEN PEPPER	Rich in vitamin C
GREENS (COLLARD, KALE, MUSTARD, TURNIP)	Calcium, cancer-fighting properties
MUSHROOMS	Good source of B vitamins, promotes healthy skin and vision, cancer-fighting properties
ONIONS	Heart-healthy compounds
PEAS	Antioxidants, compounds that play key roles in healthy vision
POTATOES	High in potassium, fiber, and vitamin C
PUMPKIN	Loaded with vitamin A, good fiber source
RADISHES	Cancer-fighting properties
RED PEPPER	Double the vitamin C of green pepper, loaded with vitamin A
ROMAINE LETTUCE	High in vitamin A and folic acid
SPINACH	Loaded with antioxidants, high in vitamin A and folic acid
SQUASH	Packed with vitamin A, good dose of calcium
TURNIPS	Fiber, cancer-fighting properties
ZUCCHINI	Good source of potassium

FRUIT	WHY WE NEED IT
APPLES	High in fiber
APRICOTS	Lots of Vitamin A
BANANAS	Potassium, fiber
BLACKBERRIES	High in fiber
CANTALOUPE	High in vitamin C and beta-carotene
CHERRIES	Heart-healthy properties
GRAPEFRUIT	High in vitamin C
GRAPES (PURPLE)	Heart-healthy properties
KIWI	Loaded with vitamin C, high in fiber
ORANGE JUICE	Terrific source of folic acid, high in vitamin C
ORANGES	Packed with vitamin C, folic acid, and calcium
PRUNES	High in fiber
RASPBERRIES	High in fiber and vitamin C
RED GRAPEFRUIT	Loaded with vitamin A
STRAWBERRIES	Rich in vitamin C, good fiber source

MEAT/EGGS	WHY WE NEED IT
BEEF (FLANK OR ROUND STEAK)	Great source of protein, iron, and B vitamins
CHICKEN BREAST (SKINLESS)	Good protein source, high in vitamin B
EGGS (WHITES)	High source of non-fat protein
TURKEY BREAST (SKINLESS)	Good protein source, high in vitamin B

GRAINS/LEGUMES/ SOY PRODUCTS	WHY WE NEED IT
BEANS (BLACK, KIDNEY, LIMA, NAVY, WHITE)	High in fiber and iron
RICE (BROWN)	Excellent source of complex carbohydrates, protein, and fiber
SOYBEANS (EDAMAME)	Excellent source of protein, fiber, iron; can reduce the risk of heart attack
TOFU	High protein source, rich in minerals, low in saturated fats, and cholesterol-free

DAIRY	WHY WE NEED IT
SKIM MILK (FAT-FREE)	High in calcium and vitamin D
YOGURT (PLAIN NON-FAT)	Good calcium source, boosts immunity

FISH/SEAFOOD	WHY WE NEED IT
COD	High in heart-healthy omega-3 fatty acids, selenium, and protein
LOBSTER	Selenium, copper
MUSSELS	Iron, selenium
ORANGE ROUGHY	Omega-3 fatty acids, high quality protein source
OYSTERS	Loaded with zinc
RED SNAPPER	Omega-3's, high-quality protein source
SCALLOPS	Good source of omega-3's

OILS	WHY WE NEED IT
CANOLA OIL	Rich in heart-healthy omega-3 and monosaturated fats
FLAXSEED OIL	Good source of essential omega-3 and omega-6 fatty acids, may reduce LDL (bad) cholesterol and reduce hypertension

SUPPLEMENT INTELLIGENTLY

You walk into a vitamin store and quickly become overwhelmed. What do you buy? Everything? Nothing? How do you take what you do end up buying?

You flip through a fitness magazine, and every other page has a dietary supplement ad on it, many of them filled with promises of amazing results, if—and it's a big if—you take the product that their particular company happens to sell at $75 a bottle. Is it a miracle in a bottle, or a swindle? There are so many products out there, so much contradictory information. What are you to believe?

It has been my overriding philosophy for many years that—with a few exceptions—the specialty-supplement industry (and by that I mean companies specializing not in basic vitamins and minerals, but in these trendy, quick-fix-type formulations) is selling the average consumer a bunch of vastly exaggerated promises, which come in pill and powder formulas. If there's one particular pitch that I find unsavory, it's the one that promises consumers that, if

PRIME

they take this certain supplement, they'll quickly gain lots of muscle (or lose lots of fat, or have tons of extra energy) and change their lives forever. This simply is not going to happen because of taking a pill or drinking a shake. Many in the industry play hardball against a man's insecurities. This becomes especially pernicious when a man gets a bit older and his habits start to catch up with him; he may be more easily convinced that there's a miracle in the next bottle of this week's supplement of the century.

The supplement industry is a multi-billion-dollar business—the business of convincing you that you can't live without their product, much like the car industry tries to do, and the detergent industry, and so forth. They want you—no, they need you—to buy their products, or they'll go out of business.

Many supplement manufacturers will push right up to the edge of what is legal in their advertising claims. The federal government tries to reign in the wildest, most blatantly misleading claims, but many in the industry keep discovering new techniques that promise (without really promising) those instant miracles to a public desperate for easy answers to tough problems. As with used cars: Let the buyer beware.

So let me be very clear about my beliefs here: There are no miracle supplements out there that are going to magically turn your health around.

On the other hand, there are some nutritional supplements that can be helpful for the 40+ man, addressing needs ranging from recuperation to pain relief. In addition, because most men won't get all the vitamins they need from their food, I'm going to provide some guidelines for basic vitamin/mineral supplementation. However, if you're reading this section hoping that I'll guide you to a miracle supplement that'll melt off all your fat, build up your muscles, and make your skin look like a baby's bottom, I fear I'm going to disappoint you. I will provide you with this "miracle," though: A lot of men waste tons of money on worthless supplements that do absolutely nothing for them. I hope that by clearing that up for you, I'll help you save you some time, money, and frustration.

So let's talk about two different categories of supplements here. First, I'll tell you about basic vitamins and minerals that every man should take, and what they do. Second, I'll discuss my top 10 additional supplements that may be of benefit to the 40+ man.

Vitamins and Minerals

In general, you're best off getting all of your vitamins and minerals from food sources. If you use my Clean Eating 70 Foods Chart in a balanced way, you'll be way ahead of the crowd.

That said, however, it's still important for the 40+ man to supplement his diet in a very basic way. This is one of those cases of more definitely *not* being better. You want to aim to get just enough.

That said, you should know that proper, yet surprisingly basic, vitamin/mineral supplementation has been shown to decrease, risk of certain cancers, heart disease, and circulatory diseases. Making sure that you have a proper amount of vitamins and minerals will also help your body fight off viral infections and will bolster your immune system. It should be emphasized that these health benefits will generally be subtle, not miraculous.

I recommend taking a basic, frill-free multivitamin/mineral tablet or pack each day with a meal. Your multivitamin/mineral should provide at least 100 percent of the RDA (recommended daily allowance) of all the nutrients listed on the package label.

In addition to that, there is strong evidence that a 40+ man can achieve positive results from a supplement combination known as an *antioxidant formula*, which battles against free radicals in the body.

Free radicals are chemical by-products of smoking, drinking, natural metabolic factors, and environmental pollution, and they have been linked not only to premature aging, but also to a wide variety of diseases that have a direct impact on the 40+ man, including heart disease and cancer. To make sure that the four key elements of the antioxidant formula are present every day, you should be sure to take (including the dosages in your multivitamin/mineral):

- Up to 2,000 mg. of vitamin C

- Up to 600 mg. of vitamin E

- Up to 200 mcg. of selenium

- Up to 60 mg. of beta-carotene

There is every indication that the proper daily levels of vitamin E reduce a man's risk of heart attack by up to 75 percent, that men who are vitamin C-deficient are at far greater risk of heart attacks, and that men taking the proper dosages of selenium can reduce the risk of prostate, bowel, and lung cancers by 40 to 50 percent. Beta-carotene is vital in boosting the body's immune system, especially as it ages. There is also strong evidence that the above daily dosage of vitamin E and beta-carotene (along with topical full-spectrum sunscreen) may protect against skin cancers. These are as close to miracles as one will get from dietary supplementation.

Trendy Supplements

There are dozens, perhaps hundreds, of trendy supplements out there being touted by manufacturers as miracles-in-a-pill. I've spent more than 20 years in the health industry, and beyond the basic benefits of reasonable levels of vitamins and minerals, and especially that antioxidant formulation that I wrote about just now, there are only a handful that I feel are even worth a moment of your attention. It's your money, but I'd say that, other than taking a look at the following eight products (and that's very far from an endorsement of all but the first two), you should stay away from all the rest. You won't get the results that the ads promise you.

I've listed these eight supplements, along with their pros and cons, so that you can make a reasonably informed decision as to whether or not you want to give them a try. I must add this warning: Anyone wanting to use these or any other dietary supplements (beyond basic vitamins and minerals) should become fully educated about potential positive and negative effects. You should also consult an enlightened physician (one who has some degree of knowledge about nutrition, which—believe it or not—still isn't very common among family doctors) about how the supplements fit in with any current treatments that you may be on, as there is often little known about the interactions between these items and prescription and over-the-counter medications.

These are two trendy supplements that I've added to my own program with positive results:

Glucosamine and Condroitin

This supplement combination has recently become enormously popular because it is reputed to help improve joint function and reduce and rebuild cartilage while simultaneously protecting the joints from any further damage. I first watched it work wonders on my elderly dog. His vet prescribed it when he showed signs of arthritis, and within six weeks he was running around with much less obvious discomfort. I began to use it when I started my own *Prime* program, since I had some old aches and pains from my many years of intense training. I felt a gentle sense of pain-relief after several weeks and experienced no side effects. I still take it.

Pros:

■ Widely considered safe and effective

■ A natural, non-drug remedy for osteoarthritis

■ No known side effects

Cons:

- The number of toxicity studies, with respect to long-term safety and side effects, is limited.

- Not all brands provide top quality ingredients.

- It typically requires six to eight weeks before effects are noticed.

- It requires long-term use for full, continued benefit.

Green Tea Extract

This is most often used to promote a higher rate of fat metabolism and loss, which is what I used it for. It is also considered to have a protective action on the cardiovascular system, as well as an antioxidant factor. Studies have linked it to cancer protection and to reduction of cholesterol, blood pressure, and blood sugar.

This was another supplement that I initially used during my *Prime* program. I was already doing everything else (exercise-and diet-wise) to lose body-fat, so I can only say anecdotally that it was a help in this area. It is interesting to note, however, that when I did a similar program without green tea extract, fat loss seemed somewhat slower. I like it mostly for its health benefits and now include it in my own personal antioxidant array. As you have also already read, I'm a big fan of drinking green tea throughout the day and truly believe that if there's something with genuine health benefits for the 40+ man that can be added to a diet, green tea and its supplement-form extract are it.

Pros:

- No major side effects

- Inexpensive and readily available

- Available with or without caffeine

- Increases fat oxidation

- Antioxidant catechins are linked to reduced heart disease risk

- May help inhibit cancer

- Available as an extract or beverage, making it easy for consistent consumption throughout the day

Cons:

■ Brands vary in amount of the active ingredient ECGC, and 270 mg or more per day are needed for full benefit.

■ Long-term fat-loss studies have yet to be done.

And the rest:

Ephedrine / Caffeine:

Used as a stimulant that acts on the central nervous system.

Pros:

■ Effective for appetite control

■ Stimulates metabolism

■ Sustained fat loss

■ Available without prescription

■ Inexpensive

■ Provides boost in energy for workouts

Cons

■ Ephedrine overdose can be fatal, and the FDA believes that ephedrine may be linked to several dozen deaths caused by high blood pressure leading to bleeding in the brain, stroke, or heart attack.

■ Can cause rise in blood pressure

■ May cause irritability, anxiety or sleeplessness

■ Can cause nausea

Guggulsterones (guggul gum or commiphora mukul herb)

Used to help increase thyroid function and to elevate metabolic rate.

Pros:

■ Lowers LDL cholesterol

■ No known side effects

- Claims to aid in fat loss

- Inexpensive

Cons:
- Not proven to cause fat loss

- Ineffective if dose per day is less than 60 guggulsterones (many brands offer too little)

Pyruvate

Used to increase fat loss and weight loss, improve endurance, reduce cholesterol, and serve as an antioxidant.

Pros:
- Effective in causing fat loss in obese dieters

- Considered to be nontoxic

Cons:
- Expensive

- Large doses required to achieve results

Ginkgo biloba

Used to enhance mental alertness and increase energy.

Pros:
- Natural anticoagulant (blood thinner)

- Increases blood circulation to the brain, possibly improving memory and concentration

- Possibly useful in the treatment of male impotence

- Inexpensive and easily obtained

Cons:
- Dangerous if taken in conjunction with prescription blood thinner, high-blood-pressure medication, or aspirin (when being used to prevent heart attack or stroke)

- Can cause upset stomach, headache, or allergic skin reaction

- Inconclusive scientific data showing any real benefits

Creatine

Used to enhance exercise recovery.

Pros:

- Can enhance exercise performance by boosting the body's ability to restore ATP (adenosine triphosphate) levels, which are needed to fuel muscles engaged in short-term, high-intensity exercise

Cons:

- Mixed reviews on actual usefulness, with some studies linking it to serious health problems such as seizures and tumors

- Manufacturers promise more than it probably delivers

- Turns to a metabolic waste product when mixed with fruit juice (so if you use it, mix with water)

- Can be toxic if overused (after the muscles are loaded during the first few days, the body can only use 2 to 3 grams per day)

- Can promote dehydration

- Linked to muscle cramps, strains, pulls, and diarrhea

- Some researchers believe that taking supplemental creatine can reduce the body's natural production of it

- Expensive

HMB (hydroxy-methylbutyrate)

Used as a protein-breakdown suppressor to make gains in muscle strength and lean mass associated with resistance training, and to prevent post-workout muscle-tissue breakdown.

Pros:

- Preliminary research (one study) seems to support the claim that HMB has an anticatabolic effect on the muscles.

- This same study shows HMB to positively affect athletic performance.

Cons:

- Often falsely promoted as something the human body doesn't produce naturally (it does—HMB is a metabolite of the amino acid leucine and is produced naturally by the human body)

- Some manufacturers claim that HMB cannot be found in food sources (it can—in catfish and grapefruit, for example).

- Supplementation means risk of upsetting the natural balance of HMB in the body.

- Very limited research available despite some manufacturers claims that it is the "next big thing." Sparse available research is conflicting regarding effectiveness.

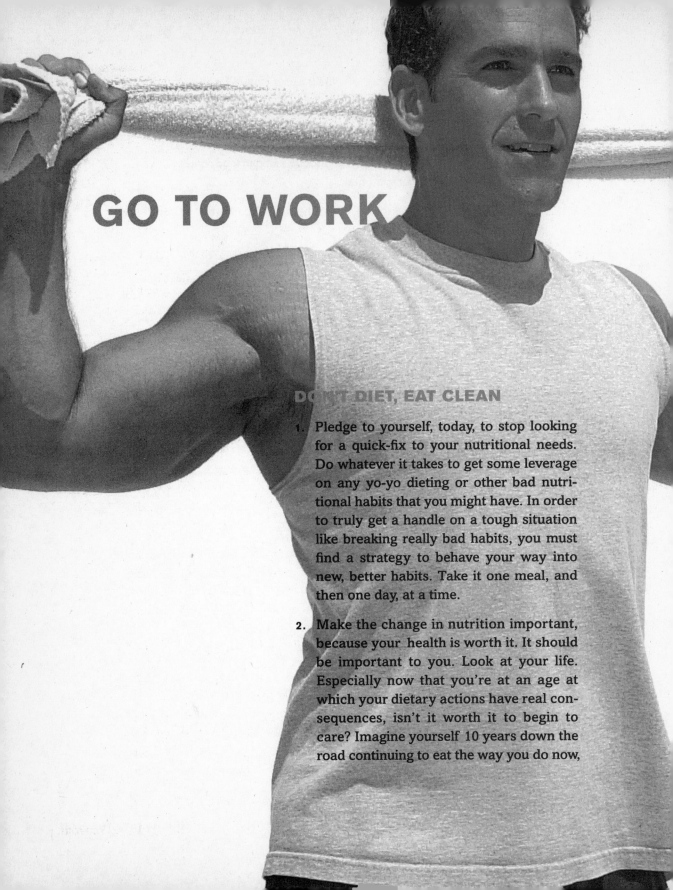

GO TO WORK

DON'T DIET, EAT CLEAN

1. Pledge to yourself, today, to stop looking for a quick-fix to your nutritional needs. Do whatever it takes to get some leverage on any yo-yo dieting or other bad nutritional habits that you might have. In order to truly get a handle on a tough situation like breaking really bad habits, you must find a strategy to behave your way into new, better habits. Take it one meal, and then one day, at a time.

2. Make the change in nutrition important, because your health is worth it. It should be important to you. Look at your life. Especially now that you're at an age at which your dietary actions have real consequences, isn't it worth it to begin to care? Imagine yourself 10 years down the road continuing to eat the way you do now,

without making any improvements (assuming a poor diet). What is your health like after those ten years? How is your weight? Are you happy with what you imagine?

3. Listen to the dialogue that you carry on in your mind about yourself. What do you say? Do words like *worthless* or *fat* or *old* come to mind; do you tell yourself that it's useless, or that your whole family is like this, all the time eating the most unhealthy diet imaginable? Go straight to those things that you say to yourself. Now is the time to redouble your efforts toward affirmations, discussed in the MOTIVATED MIND section. Take charge of your own mind today.

4. Make your eating style a priority. You'll give the most energy to the things that you find important. Plan your meals ahead of time. Make meals in advance and freeze them to zap later in the microwave. You will make the effort, if you find ways to make it more essential to your life than the old way of doing things.

5. Resist the pressure of those around you. When you make a significant change, there will be people in your life—trust me on this—who will do everything imaginable to undermine your efforts. The techniques that they use will be as varied as human personalities can be. Some will try to tempt you with goodies ("Oh, I baked this pie just for you!"). Some will offer dietary advice that's pure, uninformed hogwash. Others will be mad at you for changing. The underlying aspect about all of this is that many times, those around us don't want us to change. Often those who are trying to "help" you or who get mad at you for rejecting their cooking simply don't want to face the need for change in their own lives, and they need your agreement. Stick to your guns. You are working to make yourself healthier. That's more important.

6. When you're eating, sit down, relax, and focus on your meal. Bring your full attention to what you are eating, bite by bite. Unconscious eating (and, on the whole, unconscious living) is your enemy. Don't eat on the run. Don't eat while driving or talking on the phone. Don't eat in front of the TV. Don't eat in any circumstance where you can look up and suddenly wonder where all your food went. To make your new eating habits stick, make the meal the focus.

7. Find the leverage to break the junk-food habit. If you have to, see that burger joint or doughnut shop as an ex-smoker sees a pack of cigarettes. They're always there, no one can keep you from buying them but you—and you choose not to. The smoking/junk food comparison is more real than you might know right now. Give yourself a few months of Clean Eating, and you'll know what I mean. Just as the ex-smoker's health begins to clear with time, so too will your health improve with distance from the junk.

8. Don't allow yourself to go more than four hours without a meal (other than while you're sleeping, of course). The hunger and drop in blood sugar will create a situation that will make every drive-thru window scream out your name. Carry a meal with you. Make it a major priority.

9. Unless you're starting out seriously overweight, focus more on the health improvements that Clean Eating will bring. Stick to those 70 foods, in the right portions, with regular meals, and the excess weight will come off organically—especially when you blend it all with one of the *Prime* exercise routines.

10. Never neglect hydrating your body. You should be drinking a large glass of water every waking hour. Your body will adapt to the new water levels, and that constant need to go to the restroom will pass as it adapts. Keeping a constant flow of water is one of the fundamental ways of preventing premature aging.

EAT THESE 70 CLEAN FOODS

1. Aside from using the foods on the Top-10 list on a very regular basis (I use almost all of them daily), you should be constantly rotating the other 60 foods in your meals. Your body needs variety and should not be given exactly the same meals every day.

2. Never deep-fry, sauté in butter (or oil outside your portion), lard, or use any cooking technique that adds to the fat levels of the foods you eat.

3. Don't search for loopholes and exceptions that can be exploited in the Clean Eating plan. After all, if you find ways to cheat the system, you only cheat yourself.

4. Use healthy cooking methods when preparing your food: steaming, baking, broiling, grilling, skillet cooking with non-stick spray.

5. Make sure to use the portion guidelines listed in the Rules. If you find that you aren't getting enough food, add one more regular meal to your day and space the meals closer together.

6. Even though the oils listed are healthy, they should only be used sparingly. I give the portion as 1 tablespoon per day. Try to stick close to that. The flaxseed oil should not be heated (as with cooking). You will also note that avocado is included. While this does have great qualities, the portion should be limited to no more than 2 tablespoons every few days.

7. If you break your Clean Eating plan, don't panic and quit. Simply get back on it the next day. Your effort is what counts.

8. Remember that it takes time to adjust to any new habit. Give yourself at least three weeks to adjust. Your body will begin to respond within that time, and you'll have invested in making your efforts stick.

9. If you must "cheat," plan one day of the week (after no less than three weeks on the program) and have one meal off-diet. Then get right back on your Clean Eating plan the next meal.

10. Realize that this plan isn't just about losing weight; it's a method of transforming your health. Make the investment.

SUPPLEMENT INTELLIGENTLY

1. Always take your vitamin/mineral supplement with a meal. Usually, just before I take my first bite of breakfast, I'll take my pills.

2. If you're taking additional antioxidants, take any additional dosages at your third meal of the day. If your vitamin dosages are too high, you will simply urinate the extra out. If you break it up—especially with vitamin C—your absorption rate will be better.

3. If you decide to experiment with any of the eight additional supplements I've listed, go by the six-week rule: Invest in enough of the product for six weeks (at manufacturer's-label dosages) and take it as directed. You will need to pay attention, because supplement benefits are subtle. If you notice change—given that every other aspect of your program is on track—then it works for you and may be worth your continued use. If not, don't waste any more money.

4. Keep your vitamins and other supplements in a cool, dark cabinet. Keep track of the expiration dates on the bottles and toss them when their dates have passed.

5. I realize that I said this before, but it bears repeating: If you're on any medication at all, check with your doctor before starting any supplement course (beyond basic vitamins/minerals).

6. Be realistic with your belief system whenever you see ads for the new-new miracle. Chances are, it will be just another exaggerated claim for a supplement

that nobody will even remember in five years. If it sounds too good to be true, it probably is.

MAKE SMART ADJUSTMENTS

As you work to create new nutrition habits, you'll discover new things every day about how you approach food and meals. If you pay attention to the feedback that your body gives you, adjustments can be made every step of the way.

You should be using your journal to keep track of the meals you eat—the days where you stick with your Clean Eating, as well as the days that you might stray. Important lessons come from each notation. This is a learning process, as well as an investment in your long-term health and wellness. Paying attention will make all the difference between frustration and progress.

As you look to make personalized adjustments, ask yourself some key questions:

- Are there any areas of nutrition that need more attention?

- Am I on or off track in my efforts?

- Can I be more diligent in building my meals around the Clean Eating lists and portions?

- Have I been observing the rules of Clean Eating on a daily basis?

- Am I taking my vitamins regularly?

- Do I drink enough water?

As you did for MOTIVATED MIND and FIT BODY, go now to your journal and take a few quiet minutes to relax, focus, and review the goals that you set for your nutrition habits.

Remember to be flexible. Make adjustments. Go back and reread the sections in this book that cover areas where your progress may be lacking.

PRIME

PART FIVE

GREAT LOOKS

Destiny is no matter of chance. It is a matter of choice:
It is not a thing to be waited for, it is a thing to be achieved.

—WILLIAM JENNINGS BRYAN

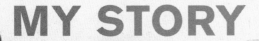

MY STORY

I grew up in a rural area. My male ancestors were farmers, carpenters and blacksmiths— hardworking men of their times. In their days, men weren't supposed to worry about how they looked; they were just supposed to accept the weathering of age and the elements and get on with life.

Besides living in a completely different era—one that is now beginning to give men tacit permission to care about their looks—I haven't really had the option of allowing time and the elements to ravage the way I look. I've made my living, to some degree, from my looks, having spent a great deal of time in front of cameras since I was 21 years old, first as a champion bodybuilder and then as a model and public personality. I have had little choice but to take care of my outward appearance. I don't consider myself a vain person. I'm actually quite low-key about my appearance. But if I was in the public eye, I couldn't allow my appearance to go to pieces.

I admit that for many years—even as I took good care of the skin on my face and body, protected myself from sun damage, looked after my hair, and so forth—at some level I couldn't help feeling that putting effort into such "superficial" matters was pretty silly. This was clearly a carryover from my ancestors' point of view. Our culture has changed since their time, however. As men, we are beginning to understand that the care we take of ourselves reflects a great deal more than good skin or hair. What I've found is that through taking care of my appearance, by doing such simple things as protecting my face from too much sun, I have benefit both my physical and mental health. In addition, in an age when most of us no longer work the fields to put food on the table, we are released from old ways of doing things—not to become vain or conceited, but rather simply to allow our self-care to be reflected in various aspects of our lives.

While I used to feel kind of funny for paying attention to how the skin on my face was doing, I don't think like that anymore. By taking care of my skin, hair, and so forth, I have kept myself looking young. Now, by looking young I don't mean that I think I appear to be 19. I wouldn't want to even if I could. I enjoy being a grown-up man. What I mean by "looking young" is that I look as if I haven't given up, or given in to what many men believe is inevitable but pray is not: hoping that some magic will happen so that they don't turn into wrinkly old men before their time.

I choose to do more than blindly hope. I choose action. I choose to set aside what previous generations thought of men caring about their looks. I've come to believe that it's irrelevant whether or not the previous generations of my male ancestors would consider my efforts to take care of my appearance to be silly. I've broken free of imagining or caring what any other person (alive or dead) might think of my efforts.

The important thing is, I care. I don't obsess; I'm not fixated; the things I do for my looks are simple and easy to do. But I care enough about myself to turn them into positive habits. I won't allow myself to grow old without a fight.

Working through the interconnected aspects of developing a MOTIVATED MIND, a FIT BODY, and SOUND NUTRITION will help the 40+ man to look and feel his best. In addition to those things, however, there are also some fairly simple steps that every man can take to assure himself of his ultimate GREAT LOOKS.

SKIN CARE

The skin that you live inside is the largest organ of your entire body. It is also the one that will show off your age to the world every bit as much as your waistline does. Just as when we see someone with a big gut we think *out of shape*, so too when we see someone with prematurely wrinkled skin we think *old*.

While there is nothing you can do about time passing and the years accumulating, there is a lot that you can do about the way your skin on your face and body looks and feels. Also, taking good care of your skin is about more than appearance. Because your skin is one of the key places where the environment meets your body, taking informed care of it can also improve your overall health.

Here are my own simple steps for achieving young and healthy skin:

Develop a Daily Routine

One of the key reasons that a man's face ages poorly is because most of us weren't raised with the habit of simple face care. It simply was considered unmasculine. I ask you to set any and all of those notions aside. If you think that your friends will give you a hard time if they know you take care of your skin, I have two suggestions:

1. Since you're reading this book, you're probably at least 40. Isn't it time to stop caring what your friends think?

2. Failing that . . . just don't tell them. Keep it your secret and you'll just look young as they wither.

Seriously though, if you follow these simple recommendations, you'll keep old Father Time from ravaging your beautiful mug. Having great-looking skin is really quite simple, but it will take some informed effort on your part.

Build the habit of doing three simple things twice each day, morning and night:

1.   Cleanse

2.   Tone

3.   Moisturize

Does it sound like a lot to do twice each day? It should only seem that way when you first start out. Then the habit will build, and it'll become second nature, especially after you see how much better you look. Besides, I've timed my routine, which I now look at as being as important as brushing my teeth. It takes a grand total of three minutes, if I do it slowly.

Every morning and night I:

1.   Completely wet my face with warm water and then gently massage a moderate amount of cleanser all over—avoiding the tender skin just under my eyes. I rotate my fingertips (or a soft-bristled complexion brush) in small circular motions and then rinse thoroughly.

2.   Then wet a cotton ball (or makeup-removal pad) with a moderate amount of toner (or astringent), and wipe all areas of my face (again avoiding the area just under the eyes). This step removes all cleanser residue that the water didn't rinse off.

3.   Finally, put a small (no larger than a dime) amount of moisturizer in the palm of one hand, wet the other hand under the tap, and then spread the water and moisturizer evenly over my face. It's important to note that moisturizer on dry skin is practically useless. The very function of a moisturizer is to trap water against the skin, and as such is a vital step for keeping skin younger-looking.

And that's it. You don't need fancy products for this routine. Stick with the basics, which you can purchase at any drugstore. You should look for products that are non-allergic. Also, do yourself a favor and buy products made for facial skin. Products such as deodorant soap and body moisturizer aren't going to do the trick—they're far too harsh and heavy. Your face has special needs.

Also, don't neglect the skin on your body when it's time to moisturize. The best time to do so is the moment that you step out of the shower, while you're still wet. Spread a small amount of moisturizing lotion everywhere. I like to use a moisturizer with aloe and vitamin E. Expensive brands are unnecessary. All you want to do is trap water against the skin. Let your skin air-dry as you continue to get ready.

Then Do This Every Week

Beyond the above three-step facial routine—performed twice every day—I also take two additional important steps that help keep my skin healthy and glowing. The main thing that makes the skin on your face appear dull or lifeless is an accumulation of dead skin cells. The cells of your skin are constantly dying off and renewing themselves. This process is known as the skin's "transit time"; in other words, the time it takes for the layers of skin to completely renew themselves. As you age, the transit time of skin-cell renewal slows considerably. We want to do what's in our power to gently speed up the rate of cell turnover and get rid of the dead surface cells. Daily washing will help, but you need more. Here's what I do to get great results:

1. Twice each week, I'll exfoliate. This is a process of scrubbing away the dead skin cells through a more vigorous cleansing. I use a product that has a grainy texture. There are many commercial facial scrubs, and a small amount of dry oatmeal grains mixed with your regular face wash will work, too. With a complexion brush (which you can buy at most drug stores) and in place of my evening cleansing (twice each week), I'll gently wash with a scrub. I won't push or scrub hard with the brush and grains; just with enough light pressure to invigorate the skin surface and *gently* exfoliate those old surface cells. You shouldn't approach this as if you're trying to sand a piece of wood. Again, be gentle!

2. Once each week, I'll give myself a cleansing mask. After I've cleansed (usually in the evening when I'm able to relax), I'll spread the goopy, wet mask over my face (avoiding the tender eye areas) and then sit back, relax (I usually meditate and visualize), and let the mask completely dry. Then I'll rinse it off, and tone and moisturize as usual. It makes the skin feel and look amazing.

And Then Once a Month

I recommend having a professional facial every month or two. The benefits are wonderful. A good facialist will completely clear your skin of dead cells and clean out all pores and impurities. Also, if you find the right spa or salon, the facialist will likely provide a very relaxing and pampering environment in which you can lie back, unwind, and let the stress of the world leave your face and your mind.

Don't Get Burned

In addition to the basics of skin care to help a man look his best—which, although it does assist in the mental health of a positive self-image, isn't totally necessary from a health perspective—there is one aspect of skin care at the center of a man's good health. That's his approach to the sun.

Aside from smoking, there's no other single way to make your skin grow old and wrinkled-looking faster than overexposure to the sun's burning rays. This point cannot be overemphasized: *There is no such thing as a healthy tan.* Tanning is, by its very nature, skin damage. Eighty percent of all skin aging results from the damage of sun exposure, and that damage will continue to build and accumulate with the passage of time. In fact, you might not even see the damage of today's sun abuse for several years, but it will likely catch up with you. And this process isn't just about looking good today; it's about setting yourself on a course to look great for years to come. You've got to think beyond today's deep tan to tomorrow's negative results.

Besides causing severe wrinkles, sun abuse also causes skin cancer, which has now grown into something of an epidemic in our culture. Between melanomas and basal-cell carcinomas, the damage of sun abuse proves that we can no longer pretend that lying around catching rays is in any way healthy.

Does the sun feel good on the skin? Yes, it does. That's simply going to have to be chalked up as one of the perverse ironies of life. The bottom line is, if you want to avoid skin cancer and keep your skin from looking 70 when you're 50, you must adjust to reality: It feels good, but if you're unprotected, it is quite bad for you.

This doesn't mean, however, that you must lock yourself in a basement. There are steps that you can take to keep having an active outdoor life.

1. Always use sunscreen. You should be wearing a minimum of SPF 15 on your face and any exposed parts of your body anytime you're outdoors. I'm never without an SPF of 30, especially when I'm at my desert house. Any sunscreen that you use should protect you from both UVA and UVB rays. Also, don't let a cloudy sky lull you into a false sense of security. The sun's rays still come through those clouds and have much of the same damaging impact on your skin. Reapply your sunscreen every few hours, after vigorous activity or after going in water.

2. Wear a broad-brimmed hat (like a floppy golf hat or straw cowboy hat) and sunglasses (preferably a wraparound style) when you go outside to further protect your vulnerable facial skin.

3. Stay out of the peak sun. Try to plan outdoor activities to avoid the most intense part of the day (between 11 A.M. and 2 P.M.).

4. Reapply sunscreen every couple of hours. In spite of what labels might say, sunscreens do wear off—even those designed for sports, water, and so forth. Go the extra mile to keep yourself healthy.

If You Want a Tan

If you still want to maintain the beach-tan look, without having to worry about cancer and deep wrinkles, get your bronze glow from a bottle. One of the side benefits of the realization that outdoor sun exposure is so dangerous has been a marked improvement in the quality of self-tanning products. However, this is one area where a little bit goes a long way.

1. Don't try to look as if you just returned from three weeks on a Hawaiian beach. The more moderate the color change you aim for, the more natural it can look. We all know what someone with way too much bronzer on looks like. Don't imitate that guy.

2. Choose a product that's right for your own needs. The stores are full both of bronzers (which color the skin temporarily and wash off) and of self-tanners (which trigger a darkening that takes some time and generally lasts a few days). Don't get caught up in the fancy-label game. All the drugstore-level tanning-product brands have good products available.

3. For your face: Wash, exfoliate, and tone first, and then apply a tanning product sparingly on the areas where the sun would naturally hit—the forehead, cheek bones, nose. Spread it on evenly, and then wash your hands completely, unless you want dark-brown palms.

4. For your body: Wash and exfoliate your skin. Spread the product on evenly, and have someone help you with hard-to-reach places. Allow it to dry before putting on any clothes that you don't want stained. Wash your hands thoroughly after the application.

5. After a few days, exfoliate the residue away and, if you want, repeat the process.

6. Remember that having a self-tanner or bronzer on is not the same as having a real tan. There is no sun protection (unless the product specifies its SPF factors on the label). Always use additional sunscreen on top of the coloring.

What About Wrinkles?

There are literally thousands of products being marketed as wrinkle solutions that claim to have anti-aging properties. In the marketing of skin products, the term "anti-aging" is something of a misnomer because, although a product may reduce the amount of damage done to your skin (as with full spectrum SPF factors), and some products may improve your skin's overall appearance (by speeding up the natural cell transit time and by moisturizing), there isn't an over-the-counter product available that can actually reverse the aging of the skin or alter the structure of the skin (if one did, it would be classified by the FDA as a drug instead of a cosmetic). It is important to note that manufacturers can label a product "anti-aging" simply by adding sunscreen to it (which, oddly, can seem both accurate and somewhat deceptive).

As with dietary supplements, all supposed wrinkle-reducers and anti-aging products should come with a bold BUYER BEWARE notice, because there are absolutely no cosmetics that function in a direct anti-aging capacity. There are, of course, surgical procedures that can reduce facial lines and wrinkles, but we're talking *surgery* here, with all the risk and expense involved, simply to remove a few lines from your face. And surgery doesn't stop the aging process. More subtle options include the use of more advanced cosmetic products; just don't be fooled by outlandish marketing or packaging. Instant youth in a bottle simply doesn't exist. There are, however, a handful of product additives that can enhance skin quality to some degree. None of them prevents or reverses the aging process. Anyone who tells you otherwise is lying.

That doesn't mean that you shouldn't use some of these more advanced products, which are certainly options for men looking to go a step or two beyond basic skin care. It's simply wise to be fully informed about what these various ingredients are and what they are actually capable of doing. Most products that claim to have anti-aging properties contain weak acids that cause the skin's outer layer to peel, thereby improving the superficial skin texture and appearance. The top four ingredients to look for are:

Alpha-Hydroxy Acids (AHAs)

Found on the labels of products ranging from face wash to moisturizers, this widely used term describes a variety of acids used to treat the skin. (The most common are *glycolic acid*, derived from the sugar cane plant, and *lactic acid*, derived from sour milk.) AHAs retexturize the skin by gently exfoliating (again, the process of shedding the surface skin) while moisturizing the new layers, and are used to treat fine lines and surface wrinkles, to improve skin texture and tone, and to unblock and cleanse pores and improve skin condition in general. While the law states that cosmetics must list ingredients on outer packaging, be aware that manufacturers are not required to note the AHA concentration and pH (acidity) levels, and your skin's response will depend on the type and concentration of the AHA (up to 10 percent), pH, and other active ingredients. (Solutions of 20 percent and stronger are considered "minipeels" and are for use by trained cosmetologists.) Also, AHA is a skin-treatment product and not a sunscreen, so if you use AHAs, even if the product has an added SPF, use additional sunscreen (at least SPF 15), as this treatment, in addition to possibly causing mild irritation, stinging, blistering, and burns (depending on concentration), can make skin more sun-sensitive.

Beta-Hydroxy Acids
These generally come in the form of salicylic acid and are used to help lighten brown spots and to lightly exfoliate. They aren't as harsh as AHAs and are available in up to a 2 percent concentration with a doctor's prescription.

Vitamin C Products
Vitamin C, a natural antioxidant, supports the formation of collagen (the connective tissue that gives skin its texture and tone) and elastin (a protein similar to collagen that is the main constituent of the skin's elastic fibers) when they've been damaged by free radicals (which result from exposure to sunlight, smoke, and pollution). Vitamin C is unstable, which means that it can easily be broken down and loses its potency quickly when exposed to air and light. Check the product label for Vitamin C in its L-ascorbic acid form, and keep the product capped tightly and stored in a cool, dry place in order to maximize its shelf life.

Retinol (Vitamin A)
Vitamin A is an antioxidant used by the body to form healthy new tissue and skin. A product designed for skin treatment that uses Vitamin A to lessen the development of new wrinkles is known as retinol and is available over the counter. The prescription version, known as tretinoin, is used to fight wrinkles and acne. These products can cause irritation and make the skin more sensitive to the sun, and therefore they should be used only in conjunction with SPF 15 or greater.

When using any of these products, in conjunction with the daily, weekly, and monthly routines outlined earlier, you may see subtle results only as long as you continue to use the product. And please remember that nothing will more effectively keep your face from getting wrinkled than proper sun protection combined with great nutrition, plenty of water, exercise, rest, and relaxation.

Additional Procedures

I've never used any of the following procedures, and this is by no means an endorsement of any kind. In fact, my sense is that most of these provide only temporary solutions and simply play on a man's insecurities. Given the dizzying array of products and treatments offered these days, this is by no means an exhaustive list but instead focuses on the most common procedures currently in use. In order to minimize potential physical and emotional scars, always be realistic about your expectations; thoroughly discuss all the pros and cons of any procedure; choose a qualified, licensed, proficient physician (or licensed professional for non-medical treatments); understand the risks, healing and recuperation times, and costs before making any final decisions.

Intense Procedures

- Dermabrasion: Performed by a surgeon under local anesthesia, this procedure can improve heavily aged skin, smooth out fine wrinkles, or improve facial scarring left from acne or an accident, through a method of controlled surgical scraping. The goal is to enhance appearance and consequently self-confidence, but dermabrasion will not remove all scars and flaws or prevent aging. And, like all surgical procedures, it is not without risk—such as of permanent darkening or blotching of the skin, development of scar tissue, or tiny whiteheads that may have to be surgically removed.

- Micro-dermabrasion (Power Peel): Requiring no anesthesia or recovery time, this technique is used to remove dry, dead, or redundant skin cells, thereby stimulating the production of young skin cells and collagen. By using abrasive mineral crystals (corundum powder), the procedure aims to improve aging skin (fine lines, brown spots) and acne (scars, blemished skin, congested skin). It may cause peeling and a sense of tightness, redness, and swelling.

- Chemical Peel: This is used to improve and smooth the texture of the facial skin by removing damaged outer layers. It can be helpful for individuals with blemishes, wrinkles, and uneven skin pigmentation, but it does not prevent or slow the aging process. The peel is made up of phenol, trichloroacetic acid and alpha-hydroxy acids specific to each individuals needs. Performed in a surgeon's office or medical facility, this is normally a safe procedure when done by a qualified, experienced plastic surgeon. However, there is always risk involved, and, in some cases, infection and scarring can occur.

- ■ Botox: This is a purified protein toxin, produced by the botulism bacteria, that is used in small, safe amounts as a wrinkle treatment. Botox is commonly used to decrease frown lines, forehead lines, and crow's feet. A small amount is injected into the muscle that creates the wrinkle. By blocking the nerve impulse from reaching that specific area (or line) the injected botox relaxes the muscle under the skin, which causes the wrinkle to soften and, at times, to disappear. Botox treatment is not permanent and typically lasts three to five months before another injection is required. (The interim is longer after several treatments.) When administered by an experienced health-care professional, it is considered safe, has no permanent side effects, and has been used in wrinkle treatment for years.

Plastic Surgery

Cosmetic surgery used to be a medical area dominated by female patients. In recent years, the number of men going under the plastic surgeon's knife has grown exponentially. Considering the fact that the overwhelming majority of plastic surgery is done for purely aesthetic purposes, it is important to enter into any procedures with eyes wide open (so to speak).

I'll be frank: I'm not a big cosmetic-surgery fan. I feel that much of the time, the patient asks for too much work to be done and has unreasonable expectations of amazing, transforming results. I've also seen way too much bad, overreaching cosmetic surgery create a growing population of men and women who have quite literally ruined their looks by buying into the silly notion that there's something wrong with the aging process (beyond what proper self-care will hold at bay) or that a particular feature doesn't match the artificial ideas of beauty shown on TV or in magazines. Most men would be far better off spending time taking care of themselves, and especially learning to like themselves, than believing that their life can be changed by having some fat sucked out (or whatever). Once again, there are no miracles out there that will replace the need to exercise, eat right, and develop a positive outlook—none.

On the other hand, some men—if they're doing all the other work on wellness and positive self-image—may find benefit from having subtle work done by a highly skilled surgeon. Do you notice that I heavily emphasize the word *subtle*.

If you go overboard, you'll end up looking like a fake, stretched-out freak. Most of us can spot horrendous plastic surgery on others; assume that others will be able to spot it on you as well, should you choose to go overboard.

Without providing an endorsement of any of the following, I'll describe the most popular procedures that men are asking for (You might notice that I don't include any of the implant procedures, such as chest, calf, and penis, because they are simply so outrageously ridiculous—and possibly dangerous—that they should be avoided at all costs):

- Face-lift (rhytidectomy): Although the face-lift is the third most desired facial plastic surgery in the United States, it should never be entered into lightly, given the seriousness of the procedure and the expense of having it done. The goal of a face-lift is to improve overall appearance, but it cannot stop the aging process. A face-lift can provide one with a more youthful appearance *if* one is in good health, has realistic expectations and has a skilled, experienced surgeon. Typically, an incision begins in the area of the temple hair, slightly above and behind the ear, before returning to the point of origin in the scalp. At that point, the skin is raised outward before the surgeon repositions and tightens the underlying muscle and connective tissue. If necessary, fat and excess skin are removed before the incision is aligned to accommodate natural beard lines. The procedure typically takes between two and four hours, depending on the involvement, and recovery typically takes two to three weeks. Even the very best face-lift results in a visible scar, and once the face-lift has been completed, the aging process continues immediately.

- Liposuction (lipectomy): This is a surgical vacuuming of fat cells from the body to produce smoother contours. This is becoming increasingly common for men (typically in the abdominal and "love handles" region). There are many risks involved, ranging from nausea to life-threatening changes in heart rhythms, and there are documented cases of people going into shock, experiencing internal bleeding and, in extreme cases, dying from the procedure if too much fat or fluid is removed. There are also plenty of individuals who report high levels of success and satisfaction after having gone through the procedure, while others experience dimpled or sagging skin. Liposuction is expensive (it typically costs between $2,000 and $10,000, depending on the body part involved), and is usually performed under local anesthetic. Effects are visible immediately. It is essential to note that unless major lifestyle changes are put in place, the fat will come back. This is not a permanent way to get lean.

- Eyelid surgery (Blepharoplasty): This surgical procedure is used to correct droopy upper eyelids or permanently puffy bags under the lower lids. With the patient under a local anesthesia, the plastic surgeon removes fat (often along with excess skin and muscle) from the upper and lower eyelids. This surgery will not remove wrinkles, dark circles, or crow's feet. Minor complications may include double or blurred vision, slight scarring, temporary swelling, and the development of tiny whiteheads once sutures are removed. More extreme risk includes difficulty closing the eyes when sleeping or a pulling down of the lower lids, which requires further surgery to correct.

- Nose-reshaping (rhinoplasty): Performed under general anesthesia, this procedure is usually done to correct a deviated septum (the hole between the nostrils), correct breathing problems by widening nasal passages, or aesthetically improve the overall look of the face. The surgeon typically makes an incision under the nose, between the nostrils, in order to make changes to the cartilage and bony hump on the ridge of the nose. Side effects range from mild complaints of dry lips, difficulty swallowing, and bruising and swelling around the eyes and cheeks to serious complications such as poor cosmetic results, chronic nosebleeds, hypersensitivity, and difficulty breathing.

AND THEN THERE'S HAIR

Very few things worry men more than when they first see loose hairs coming off their heads and swirling down the shower drain. Even though it is quite normal for a man to shed up to 100 hairs each day, it still can shake the nerves. Most men who are 40+ have a pretty good idea whether or not their full head of hair is going to stick around for the ride. And, since most men will experience some form of hair loss in their lifetimes, it only stands to reason that this process should be seen as quite normal.

So, what should you do if you find yourself with less than a full head of hair? My first piece of advice is to find a way to relax. There's nothing you can do about it. By that I don't mean that there aren't tons of solutions being marketed right this minute. It's just that, no matter which of those solutions you might try, you'd still have lost much of your own natural head of hair. Think of it this way: I have brown eyes. I can wear blue contacts, but that doesn't mean that my eyes are really blue. It means that I'm trying to convince others that they are. I still know I have brown eyes—given current technology, that isn't going to change. It's much the same with hair. But I'm a big believer in finding a balance between taking great care of yourself and accepting natural traits that can't be fully changed.

As we all know, there are a lot of options out there. There are weaves, drugs, plugs, combovers, surgery, micrografts, and so forth. This is where some men will agree with me and others will think I'm crazy: I think that if your hair has thinned out, you should skip all those artificial measures and learn to accept yourself. Unless you spend upwards of $5,000 to $10,000, wigs look fake (tell me you can't spot one from a mile away) and require major maintenance, plus you walk around knowing that you're wearing a hairpiece. The surgical options are pretty frightening: They all leave major scars, and almost all forms have a very high failure rate. The drugs? Rogaine will grow a bit of fuzz, but it'll all drop away the minute you quit taking the stuff. And the fact remains that with any of these artificial measures, you'll still know what lies beneath.

Bald is beautiful. Look at Michael Jordan, Ed Harris, Bruce Willis, and so on. Accept yourself. Cut it short and be proud. But that's just one man's opinion.

If you've gone gray, my feelings are very much the same: Accept yourself. If you do feel the need to color over the gray, do yourself a huge favor and seek out the best colorist in your area. Those dyes from the grocery store—the ones that you put in over your bathroom sink—make your hair all one color. Very little looks more fake than a one-color jet-black dye job that isn't worn ironically.

To keep the hair you have on your head healthy and glowing, try these tactics:

- Unplug the blow dryer. It dries out your hair and makes it look dull.

- Realize that, with age, the hair shafts grow more fine, which makes them more fragile. The scalp also gets drier. Try baby shampoo. It's gentle and shouldn't dry you out.

- Use a hot oil treatment once a month on your freshly washed hair.

- Don't over-shampoo, unless you have very oily hair.

- Above all else, get a great haircut that's flattering and age-appropriate.

IN CONCLUSION

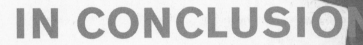

With a strong emphasis on paying attention, making informed efforts, and investing in a good dose of healthy self-regard, a man can enter into the second half of his life in amazing health and physical condition. He simply must understand what it takes to do so and be willing to make a positive investment in himself.

If I were asked to boil down all of the various elements of a *Prime* program into a ten-point cheat-sheet, it would look like this:

1. You should develop a realistic and positive attitude and self-image.

2. Become motivated to work constructively on aspects of yourself that are changeable (and that you desire to change) and become accepting of those parts of you that are unchangeable.

3. Set reasonable, sustainable goals that you review and update on a regular basis.

4. Perfect a style of physical exercise that meets your own realistic fitness needs and goals.

5. With your exercises, create a reasonable and sustainable balance of strength, endurance, and flexibility.

6. Get plenty of high-quality rest, and work to keep your reaction to life's stressors under your control.

7. Never diet again; instead, develop a workable, healthy, long-range nutrition style.

8. Take only the vitamins, minerals, and nutrition supplements that you really need.

9. Protect and care for your outer appearance, especially your skin.

10. Learn to accept the natural aging process while simultaneously working to hold it at bay.

Now, go out, take charge, and enjoy the absolute *Prime* of your life!

INDEX

PRIME

By the time Bob Paris was 23 years old, he was a Mr. America and a Mr. Universe. In a matter of four years, he had gone from being a homeless teenager to a World Champion, and he went on to become one of the most respected, celebrated, and photographed athletes in the history of bodybuilding.

Since then, he has traveled the world, speaking to groups at universities, corporations, and many more locations on topics ranging from fitness, self-improvement, and motivation to overcome adversity and developing self-esteem. He has been nominated for Lecturer of the Year on the national collegiate speaking circuit and has received recognition from many quarters for his philanthropic efforts.

Bob is the author of several books, which include the fitness titles *Beyond Built*; *Flawless and Natural Fitness*; as well as the critically acclaimed memoir, *Gorilla Suit: My Adventures in Bodybuilding*.

Visit the official Bob Paris website at: www.BOBPARIS.com